THE NATURAL WAY SERIES

Increasing numbers of people worldwide are falling victim to illnesses which modern medicine, for all its technical advances, seems often powerless to prevent – and sometimes actually causes. To help with these so-called 'diseases of civilization' more and more people are turning to 'natural' medicine for an answer. The *Natural Way* series aims to offer clear, practical and reliable guidance to the safest, gentlest and most effective treatments available – and so to give sufferers and their families the information they need to make their own choices about the most suitable treatments.

Other titles in the Natural Way *series*

THE NATURAL WAY

Chronic Fatigue Syndrome

Gill Jacobs

Series medical consultants
Dr Peter Albright MD (USA)
& Dr David Peters MD (UK)

Approved by the
AMERICAN HOLISTIC MEDICAL ASSOCIATION
& BRITISH HOLISTIC MEDICAL ASSOCIATION

E L E M E N T
Shaftesbury, Dorset ● Rockport, Massachusetts
Melbourne, Victoria

© Element Books Limited 1997
Text © Gill Jacobs 1997

First published in the UK in 1997 by
Element Books Limited
Shaftesbury, Dorset SP7 8BP

Published in the USA in 1997 by
Element Books, Inc.
160 North Washington St
Boston MA 02114

Published in Australia in 1997 by
Element Books
and distributed by
Penguin Books Australia Limited
487 Maroondah Highway, Ringwood, Victoria 3134

Cover design by Slatter-Anderson
Designed and typeset by Linda Reed and Joss Nizan
Printed and bound in Great Britain by
Caledonian International Book Manufacturing Ltd,
Glasgow

British Library Cataloguing in Publication

Library of Congress Cataloging in Publication
data available

ISBN 1 86204 113 X

Contents

List of Illustrations

Acknowledgements

Over the years many people have helped me understand Chronic Fatigue Syndrome (CFS) – not just how to interpret new research, but also what it feels like to live with this chronic and debilitating illness. Their knowledge and experience has been invaluable. I would like to thank them all, including staff and members of Action for ME and Chronic Fatigue, the members of the ME/CFS Charities Alliance (UK), Fiona Agombar, Martin Arber, Dr Veronica Beechey, Leon Chaitow, Jane Colby, Sue Finlay, Clare Francis OBE, Dr Alan Franklin, Dr Ellen Goudsmit, Dr Anne Macintyre, Dr Sarah Myhill, Alf Riggs, Dr Pat Shipley and Ondine Upton. They may not all agree with everything I say, but their patience, advice, insights and experience proved invaluable.

Clare Watson's contribution to a paper on Chronic Fatigue (D Peters, *Complementary Therapies in Medicine*, 1996, 4), where she talks about the psychodynamic approach, as a recovered PWC (person with CFS) and a clinical psychologist, was invaluable. She addresses the psychological needs of both the patients with CFS and those trying to help them. She also clarified the notion that a refusal to acknowledge the emotional consequences of chronic illness, by both the doctor and the patient, can impede recovery.

Thanks too to the Yoga for Health Foundation for allowing me to experience their gentle way with CFS, and the many contributors to Action for ME's journal, *InterAction*, who, in a variety of ways demonstrate that there is no one way to recover from this complex and baffling illness.

Foreword on the use of
the name for the illness

The use of the term Chronic Fatigue Syndrome (CFS) for
this book refers to what is sometimes known in Great
Britain as ME or Myalgic Encephalomyelitis. Whilst
patient support groups argue that 'ME' should be
retained to denote a separate disease process, CFS is
the label preferred by doctors in Great Britain. As used
by them, it refers to a whole spectrum of fatigue states
and causes.

CFS is the term most used in the USA by scientists,
with some patient groups using alternatives such as
CFIDS (Chronic Fatigue Immune Deficiency Syndrome).
This highlights the differences between themselves
and other fatigue states without problems of immune
function.

While the jury is still out about a name which is
acceptable to different countries, and different groupings
within the same country, I have chosen to use CFS, in
order that this book can be addressed to both sides of the
Atlantic. I would like to point out, however, that I would
support a new name, reflecting the neurocognitive
aspects of this illness, and its distinction from 'everyday
tiredness' or 'tired all the time'.

For ease of reference, I list below the names which are
commonly used for the illness.

- Chronic Fatigue Syndrome (CFS) was originally used in Australia and the USA. More recently, it has been adopted by American and British psychiatrists as a 'convenience' umbrella term, which also covers some illnesses which are caused by psychological factors. The problem is that fatigue is not always the predominant feature. The variety of different conditions means that very different populations can be included under the one term, which means that research results are not strictly comparable. Patient groups throughout the world are unanimous in their view that chronic fatigue syndrome does not describe the symptoms and resulting disability.

- PWC is a shorthand term for 'people with chronic fatigue syndrome', and as such is widely used in the USA because it avoids the use of the term 'sufferer'.

- Myalgic Encephalomyelitis (ME) was the name developed following the Royal Free Hospital outbreak in the UK in 1955. However, because the name ME does not accurately describe what happens to the body (not everyone has muscle pain, and there is still controversy about whether there is inflammation of the spinal cord and the brain) doctors in the UK now use CFS. Patient support groups agree that the term may be an incorrect description of what happens, but they prefer to use it rather than CFS because it is a convenient way to distinguish between general chronic fatigue and chronic fatigue associated with neurological symptoms.

- Post/Persistent Viral Fatigue Syndrome (PVFS) is sometimes used in the UK as a synonym for CFS. However, it is misleading because not all cases of CFS are triggered by viruses.

- Chronic Fatigue Immune Dysfunction Syndrome (CFIDS) was introduced as a reaction to the inadequacies of the term CFS, because it acknowledges the research findings which show immune dysfunction. Many PWCs prefer this term to CFS, because they claim that fatigue is not the most troublesome symptom. This term is mostly used in the USA.

- Fibromyalgia Syndrome (FMS) is coming to be seen as almost identical to CFS, and certainly related. The predominant feature is joint and muscle pain, together with the other symptoms of CFS. Both groups have reduced blood flow and energy production in key sites of the brain. For both there is no accepted single cause, and they both have chronic symptoms which include fatigue, muscle pain, neurocognitive dysfunction, mood disturbances and sleep disturbances. There are 6 million sufferers in the US.

Introduction

If you are fortunate enough not to have Chronic Fatigue Syndrome (CFS), imagine having symptoms which suddenly make you feel like a flat battery, with no easy way to get recharged. Imagine, too, the problems of having an illness which is controversial and is still being debated by doctors, who are uncertain as to the cause and even more uncertain as to treatment. And all the time you are surrounded by scepticism as to whether you are really ill, because there are no tests to prove it. More and more doctors now recognize CFS and may indeed be sympathetic. But when it comes to advice on what to do, and how to treat it, there is still a great deal of uncertainty.

Despite more and more research evidence suggesting that CFS could be a neurological disease – that is a disease of the central nervous system – there are still a number of doctors who choose to focus primarily on the fatigue. In fact the other symptoms, such as poor temperature control, extreme sensitivity to sound and light, loss of balance, loss of short-term memory and muscle and joint pain, are seen by most sufferers as even more distressing than the fatigue.

By paying less attention to these symptoms, which are hard to test for, some doctors view the illness as one which is kept going by psychological factors. They do not deny that there may have been evidence of a viral infection in the first instance, but suggest that CFS is unnecessarily prolonged by patients who have a need to hide behind their symptoms as a way of avoiding past psychological problems. In fact the major problem for those with CFS, apart from the symptoms, is their despair at not being able to get back to their former capacities.

The approach of this book is that it is more helpful to see CFS as not one but a number of different combinations of causes, leading to the same group of symptoms. Applying the psychological label, above all others, is one-dimensional and unhelpful. A holistic approach, which recognizes the interplay between physical and psychological, offers more hope for recovery.

Fortunately, there are signs of shifts towards a more balanced perspective. In 1995 the American government voted $11.8 million for wide-ranging research into the problem (thanks in part to the enormous lobbying capacity of people with CFS). In September 1996 the National Institute of Allergy and Infectious Diseases and the National Institutes of Health in the USA published a sympathetic and informative set of guidelines for physicians. One month later the Royal Colleges of Physicians, Psychiatrists and General Practitioners in the UK published a report which was more tentative in its conclusions, despite the research evidence. It did, however, acknowledge the genuine and disabling nature of the syndrome.

No one treatment has been found to work for CFS as a whole. Whilst those affected by this illness have had to fight for recognition or wait for agreement on treatment, many have quietly got on with trying to help themselves. Those who have been given drug therapy for individual symptoms have discovered that CFS does not respond well to this form of treatment, and the vacuum is therefore being filled by complementary therapies, many of which have been shown not only to improve symptoms but also to remove some of them altogether. In unravelling the puzzle of what to do there are many different routes to take, the order and combination of which are individual to each person's needs. Whatever therapy you choose, however, the self-help aspects of this illness are crucial. Energy management and pacing are vital tools to recovery, and should partner other interventions, whatever they are.

This book is an attempt to make the choices for treatment and self-help clearer and more manageable. It is also an attempt to give you the permission you need to dare to hope.

CHAPTER 1

What is chronic fatigue syndrome?

Chronic Fatigue Syndrome (CFS) is a chronic, debilitating disorder characterized by fatigue, pain and cognitive dysfunction (eg impairment of short-term memory, loss of powers of concentration, disturbed sleep patterns and emotional swings).

CFS is often thought to be merely the same as 'tired all the time' (TATT). This is far from the case. Many PWCs (people with chronic fatigue syndrome) have severe muscle aches, and other symptoms include difficulties with concentration and memory, loss of balance, digestive problems, visual disturbances, sleep disorders, poor temperature control and mood swings.

The unpredictability of symptoms, alternating hope with despair, is particularly hard to cope with. Disturbed sleep patterns, which can result in wakefulness at night and falling asleep in the day, make life even harder. The temptation, on good days, is to make up for lost time. The roller coaster of raised expectations and shattered hopes for recovery is hard to live with, and is usually brought on by overdoing things, either physically or mentally. For example, in the early stages some PWCs only have sufficient energy to brush their hair, but not enough to walk across a room. Forcing yourself against what your body is telling you to do can cause long-term damage. On the other hand, resting in order to restore energy levels seems to work in the short term, but does not cure the illness.

Symptoms of CFS

A diagnosis of CFS should be based on careful history, examination and exclusion of other conditions (*See* p7). The following characteristic features have to be present:

- an acute reaction, sometimes delayed up to 72 hours, to either physical or mental exertion, which can be trivial compared to the PWC's previous tolerance, and from which they can take many days to recover – 'healthy' fatigue, which is alleviated by rest, is not the same
- central nervous system symptoms, including poor concentration, short-term memory loss and disturbances of sensation
- variability of symptoms from day to day or within one day, which is severe enough to affect daily activities
- chronicity – a tendency to persist over months or even years

The following are not necessarily experienced by everyone with CFS, and are not essential for diagnosis, but many people have them in addition to those above:

- a viral trigger – most cases of CFS start after a viral infection
- symptoms suggestive of chronic infection – low-grade fever, tender lymph glands and sore throat, often with diarrhoea and gastric pain
- cognitive problems in addition to those above – word-finding difficulties, an inability to comprehend/retain what is read, an inability to calculate numbers and impairment of speech and/or reasoning
- muscle symptoms – exercise-induced muscle weakness, taking days to recover, an inability to stand for long periods or to raise the arms even to hold a telephone or brush one's hair, sore and aching muscles with tenderness, twitching muscles after overuse, problems with reading or writing
- autonomic disturbances – palpitations, rapid pulse, chills and night sweats, sudden pallor, poor temperature

control, nausea, diarrhoea, bladder dysfunction, hormonal disturbances
- sensory disturbances – reactions to sound, light and smells, tinnitus
- sleep disturbance – at first the need to sleep all the time, followed in the chronic stage by insomnia, loss of non-REM sleep and vivid, unpleasant dreams
- emotional fluctuations – depression, but without the usual reactions of apathy and feelings of worthlessness and guilt, irritability, anxiety, panic attacks, personality changes, mood swings
- pain – sometimes severe headache, abdominal pains, back, neck or facial pain, chest pain, joint pain with or without swelling
- gut symptoms – bloating, pain, wind, irritable bowel, food intolerance, malabsorption (not getting the goodness from the food)
- inability to tolerate alcohol – an almost universally experienced symptom
- symptoms of gut dysbiosis and fungal overgrowth – alternating diarrhoea and constipation, anal itching, thrush, bloating, wind, sugar craving, cystitis, pre-menstrual tension
- heart complications: rapid pulse, ectopic beats, angina-like chest pain
- other: weight changes without changes in diet, light-headedness, feeling in a fog, fainting

Current research on CFS is providing increasing support for the view that something is going wrong at the level of the cell. This interferes with chemical processes and the ability of cells, especially muscle and nerve cells, to produce energy and transmit messages to the brain. Research demonstrates that CFS causes particular changes in the brain, resulting from reduced blood flow in the brain stem. These changes are different from those found in depression. There are also hormonal and nervous system changes. CFS is usually triggered by a viral infection, although some people describe a slow slide into the illness, without any obvious infectious trigger. The often severe cognitive complaints distinguish CFS from other, similar disorders.

Up to 20 per cent of sufferers become permanently disabled, although these figures may reflect the consequences of bad management in the early stages if CFS is poorly understood. Of the remainder, a minority manage to return to normal life after one or two years. The majority, however, have to live with CFS for a number of years; there is a lot of uncertainty about how to help yourself, whilst conventional medicine still debates causes as opposed to treatment. In fact, early and accurate diagnosis, with appropriate energy management and a holistic perspective, greatly reduces the chances of permanent disablement.

CFS: a 20th century disease?

Although the terminology for these conditions is comparatively new, the disorders themselves are not. Thomas Sydenham, the father of English medicine, described a similar symptom pattern to CFS as muscular rheumatism in 1681. Florence Nightingale became ill after returning from the Crimean War, and spent years housebound and too exhausted to receive more than one visitor at a time. Her exposure to the risk of infection and her gruelling work schedule, which would not have allowed her to rest, suggest that she is likely to have had what we now know to be CFS. In the American Civil War CFS was recognized as 'soldier's disease', and the neurologist-in-chief for the Union Forces, Silas Weir Mitchell, published a book on the disease. He suggested total bed rest and hypernutrition for a period of several months.

The polio link

A form of CFS was recognized for the first time as a separate epidemic disease during an epidemic of polio in
California in 1934. It did not have the severe muscle
wasting found in polio, but the similarities were enough
for the term 'atypical polio' to be coined. The symptoms
were those of CFS, with relapsing muscle weakness,
unusual pain syndromes, personality changes, memory
loss, etc. In fact the majority of the 198 doctors and nurses
affected by CFS fell ill after being injected with an extract
made from the blood of those they were treating during
the epidemic, and which was intended to enhance
immunity. Most never fully recovered, although they
received substantial compensation.

According to Dr Richard Bruno, an American clinical
psychophysiologist, 91 per cent of polio survivors now
develop post-polio syndrome, many years after the initial polio, with almost identical symptoms to CFS.

Since 1934 well over 50 similar clusters or epidemics
to the one in California have appeared in the medical literature, using many different names but sharing the
same body of symptoms. But with the introduction of
polio immunization from 1953 to 1955 the paralytic form
of CFS declined, along with the incidence of polio. From
that point CFS was more usually seen in individual
cases, but typical symptoms still included headache,
muscle pain, giddiness, emotional swings, fatigue
which came and went, visual disturbances and poor
temperature control. Some doctors suggest that as polio
vaccination wiped out paralytic polio, there were worldwide epidemics of other enteroviruses (bowel viruses, of
which the polio virus is one), which then had more
chance to take hold.

Dr Melvin Ramsay was the first specialist to note that
many people contracting CFS remained ill after long

periods of time, some showing no signs of recovery at all. His involvement with CFS developed during an epidemic at the Royal Free Hospital in Britain in 1955, affecting mainly nurses. Despite obvious signs of infection, the involvement of the central nervous system and the fact that some of the victims were still disabled 15 years later, a reassessment of these cases by two psychiatrists from case-notes in 1970 came to the conclusion that they were suffering from mass hysteria. This then became the 'verdict' that continued to appear in medical textbooks. A similar situation occurred in other affected countries in the developed world.

Why do some doctors and patient groups still disagree?

Although doctors are more likely now to acknowledge an initial viral trigger rather than hysteria in the majority of cases, the fact that symptoms are prolonged is attributed by some psychiatrists who specialize in CFS to psychological causes, which need to be addressed by encouraging the PWC gradually to increase mobility. Studies conducted by these psychiatrists suggest that some PWCs, whilst genuinely ill to start with, somehow hang on to the symptoms and retreat from life as a way of avoiding psychological pain. The diagnosis of CFS shields them from the stigma of depression or neurosis. The deconditioning of unused muscles is seen as being at the core of the problem, and patients are encouraged to let go of their illness beliefs because they are inappropriate and hinder their recovery.

Patient support groups disagree with this approach, whilst acknowledging that a few people may be helped by it. They suggest that it does not address the depth and seriousness of CFS, backing up their position by quoting studies which show evidence of immune dysfunction in CFS, over and above psychological causation.

They argue that in the initial stage of the illness, before symptoms stabilize, too much exercise can cause a relapse. Certainly, there is general agreement that CFS symptoms are exacerbated by stress; the disagreements seem to revolve around whether the symptoms are prolonged merely by psychological stress, or also by profound physiological changes in the body. Time, or interventions other than just psychological, are necessary for recovery according to this holistic perspective.

The role of nutrition, the environment and chemical exposure in CFS is more likely to be considered by complementary therapies, where the understanding of the

---

Other illnesses which sometimes cause fatigue

In diagnosing CFS, the following illnesses, which can also cause fatigue, need to be excluded by thorough evaluation based on history, physical examination and appropriate laboratory findings:

- thyroid disorders
- anaemia
- Addison's disease
- cancer
- multiple sclerosis
- diabetes
- gastrointestinal disorders
- auto-immune diseases
- chronic infections such as HIV, glandular fever and tuberculosis
- toxoplasmosis
- parasites
- nutritional deficiencies
- connective tissue diseases
- psychiatric disease such as endogenous depression or anxiety neurosis
- the side effects of a chronic medication or other toxic agent such as a chemical solvent or pesticide

mind/body connection is open to the inclusion of all these factors. However, a small number of doctors are also beginning to move in this direction.

Who is most at risk and why

Estimations of the incidence of CFS vary widely in different settings depending on whether British, American or Australian case definitions are used. British epidemiologist Dr E G Dowsett notes that this is unlikely to be corrected until a common terminology and case definition is agreed worldwide.

In the US it is thought that previous estimates of the number of people with CFS had been grossly underestimated by the Centers for Disease Control. The new estimates state that there are 75–267 cases of CFS per 100,000 people in the general population. These figures were drawn from the community, however, rather than from those seeking medical help. The previous figures had only been 2.0–7.3 cases per 100,000.

In the UK it is thought that around 150,000 suffer from CFS, twice as many as Multiple Sclerosis. This figure is probably an underestimate, although it is true to say that we are entering a period of decrease, after what appears to have been an epidemic in the late 80s and early 90s. However, the Royal Colleges report estimates a prevalence figure of up to one million cases in primary care. The ME/CFS Charities Alliance considers this to be an overestimate which is not reflected in claims for sickness and disability benefits, and which demonstrates the danger of lumping together all cases of chronic fatigue, with very different causes, degrees of severity and management needs.

Patient profile

A study by Drs Darrel Ho-Yen and I McNamara of 293 CFS patients found that 64 per cent were women and 36 per cent men. However, the severity of the illness and the use of the doctor's time was the same among men and women. The largest percentage, of 29 per cent, were in the age range 35–44, and 22 per cent were teachers and students.

A peak occurs in the 20–40 age group, but children as young as 5 are affected. All socioeconomic groups are represented, although there is a strong contingent of teachers and health professionals, who are more exposed to high levels of stress at work and to the risk of infection. One of the problems with studies to assess prevalence, however is that different definitions may have been used.

Janet

Janet is a journalist in her forties. A few months before she fell ill she had damaged her knee in a road accident, which left her with a temporary limp, and also aggravated the nagging pain from an old back injury. She had had a difficult couple of years, because of her mother's death, financial worries and the end of a long-term relationship, but felt things were starting to come together.

On top of this she had been working long hours, sometimes 15 a day. Looking back now, she realizes that this contributed to the breakdown of her health, but her feeling of indestructibility at this time did not alert her to the need to cut down. The immediate trigger to her collapse was a sore throat, which she ignored in her determination to keep active at work.

She remembers the day she first became ill very clearly. She lay down and simply could not get up.

'After three hours I had to roll off the sofa, and crawl to the kitchen to make myself a drink. It was very frightening.' She collapsed when she struggled into work a few days later. Although she tried to work at home, she became more and more ill over the next three months. She remembers how she would wait to put the kettle on until she needed to go to the bathroom, because she did not have the energy to make two separate trips from her bedroom. She relied on friends and relatives to do her shopping and cook meals. Every morning, however, she forced herself to wash and dress, in an effort to lift her morale.

Her memory was so bad that she would forget which way she had been going when she paused for a rest on her way along the hall. She would have to sit down to try and remember. Apart from memory loss and extreme fatigue, which fluctuated, her symptoms included muscle and joint pain, sweaty feet, indigestion, extreme sensitivity to noise and light, and clumsiness. She was unable to watch television because she could not follow what was happening. She was hospitalized for a week when her arms and hands became too weak to move. Although her brain had 'turned to jelly', her helplessness did not leave her feeling passive – something she now finds hard to understand. She did, however, have occasional bouts of despair.

Throughout she had the support of a sympathetic doctor, who, at her request, prescribed evening primrose oil, and supported her when she tried homoeopathy and Chinese herbs. Three months on, however, her family were so worried that she was taken to live with her sister where, after a couple of months, she started to improve.

Eight months after she fell ill, she was back at work full time, but she would have a relapse every spring and autumn. After a year she admitted that she could not cope and started working at home one day a week. Her colleagues would often cover for her in order that she could spend the 'work day' resting in bed. Her last relapse was early in 1995, three years after it all began. She now works freelance from home and has fully recovered.

Janet feels that with any illness it is important to keep optimistic. It is important to find out all you can about your condition and possible remedies, but you should avoid letting health problems dominate your life. She admits that that was often an impossible target because of the distressing nature of CFS symptoms.

She believes going back to work can be helpful in the long run, once you are in the recovery phase when symptoms have stabilized, as long as you have some control over your hours, and the pace of work. Finding the right balance between pushing yourself into relapse and holding back until you slide into a downward spiral of inactivity is the key. Janet feels that her chronic back pain had taught her to put herself outside the pain and get on with her life, although this may at the same time have encouraged her not to listen to her body, which in turn could have led to her becoming ill in the first place.

CHAPTER 2

The body and chronic fatigue syndrome

CFS is a serious and complex illness that affects many different body systems. Research is beginning to confirm the likelihood of various sub-groups with different constellations of causes. Whilst the experts are debating whether the cause is primarily physical (persistent virus together with toxic damage is one of the latest theories) as opposed to psychological (depression and/or symptom dependency), we are forced to try to make sense of a myriad of research findings. Despite the problems of definitions of CFS, which vary or are too loose, some order is beginning to emerge.

It is important, when assessing the pieces from the 'physical' jigsaw, to ensure that this does not rule out the ability of the mind to contribute to the healing process. The question is whether that is enough on its own.

The immune system

The immune system is part of the body's defence against infection, although the skin, digestion and mucous membranes lining the internal organs are the first line of defence. If you are healthy, the immune system is constantly on the alert to ward off anything which might hurt or harm you.

Research evidence

● There is research evidence showing that there are problems with the way the immune system behaves.

● This can exist side by side with abnormalities in the function of the central nervous system – the brain and spinal cord.

● Linked to this, and possibly underlying both problems, is a malfunction of the hypothalamus, pituitary glands and adrenal glands – also known as the HPA axis (the system which deals with stress and emotions).

● Behind this, and coming right down to the smallest unit in the body, is the possibility of malfunction in the mitochondria, the power house of the cell.

Immune dysfunction can be caused by different factors from inherited weakness to nutritional deficiencies, infection or prolonged stress. For example, secretory IgA, part of the body's immune protection in the gut mucosa, was shown to be reduced in one study when students prepared for and took exams. It took three weeks to return to normal.

Underactivity and overactivity can occur at the same time in different parts of the immune system, and is possibly explained by the inefficiency of a system when it is continually on the alert. It is common for some PWCs not to develop colds because they cannot fight infection – catarrh or mucus production in a cold is a sign that your immune system is working to fight the infection. On the other hand, and sometimes at the same time, there is evidence of an overactive immune system in CFS because there are raised levels of cytokines (by-products of immune function) in the blood of some PWCs. Another effect of abnormal immune response is allergic reactions. Multiple allergies are common in CFS, both to different foods and to chemicals in the environment.

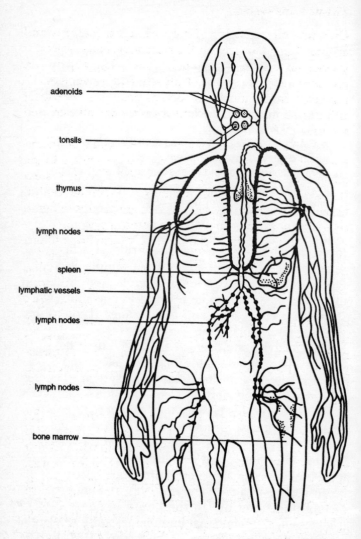

Fig. 1 The immune system

The nervous system

Our awareness, sense of self, thought, feelings and actions depend largely on the central nervous system. It is essential to sensory perception, the feeling of pain and pleasure and the control of muscle and movements. It regulates bodily functions such as breathing, heartbeat and digestion. Language and memory are also created through it.

The central nervous system is centred in the brain and the spinal cord and controls all the nervous tissue in the other parts of the body. The peripheral nervous system is made up of nerves, which connect up with the central nervous system, and ganglia, which are groups of nerve cells sited at various points in the nervous system.

The working parts of the nervous system are millions of interconnected nerve cells called neurones. Their job is to pick up signals in one part of the nervous system and send them to another, where they may be relayed on to other neurones, or to bring about some action. The central nervous system acts as a 'switchboard' for incoming and outgoing electrical impulses in order to regulate all the body's activities, including the chemically controlled ones. Vibrations from these electrical impulses help to switch on or turn off processes necessary for healthy functioning.

The hypothalamus (*see* pp18–19) controls the autonomic nervous system – breathing, heartbeat and digestion – responding to any information about variations in, for example, the body's chemical status. One example of the control of the autonomic nervous system by the hypothalamus is the increase in heart rate needed to supply more oxygenated blood when there is increased demand during exercise. The hypothalamus is also closely related to the most emotional part of the brain, the limbic system.

Studies suggest that the nervous system is involved in CFS. Experiments in mice were consistent with the notion that fatigue could be due to cytokine production within the central nervous system. Cytokines help in the task of killing infected cells, and a raised level in the blood suggests an ongoing viral infection. Furthermore, the cognitive problems associated with CFS – eg short-term memory loss, difficulty with speech, visual and spatial problems, unusual headaches, losing track of a train of thought, vivid and disturbing dreams, – could all be related to problems in the brain and the central nervous system.

The brain

Brain function directly influences immune function, either through hormones in the bloodstream or through the nerves. Neuropsychological tests on some patients with CFS have revealed abnormalities which are consistent with a brain disorder, even though they were not affected by a clinical depression.

Other studies have shown that PWCs with higher cognitive difficulty scores have more problems with immune function than those with fewer cognitive problems. Depression was not shown to be the cause. Some studies have found that cognitive functioning was impaired in patients with CFS who did not have psychiatric disease. Their conclusion was that impaired cognition in CFS cannot be explained solely by the presence of a psychiatric condition.

Some medical authorities, on the other hand, argue that severe cognitive symptoms, such as difficulties with memory, attention and concentration, demonstrate that CFS is primarily a psychological illness and so argue that psychological factors maintain it, even if there is a viral trigger.

The brain can be divided into three different regions: hindbrain, midbrain and forebrain. The cerebellum, in the hindbrain, is mainly concerned with the unconscious control of movement, sending out signals to muscles to maintain posture and balance, and coordinating body movements with the motor areas of the cerebrum. PWCs have problems with gait (walking) and move differently from others, and one of the tests for CFS uses gait.

The brain stem is particularly affected in CFS. It links the brain with the spinal cord, and comprises part of the hindbrain, all of the midbrain and part of the forebrain. All incoming and outgoing messages come together and cross over in the brain stem – they cross over because the left side of the body is governed by the right side of the brain and vice versa.

Sophisticated brain scans from several studies have shown that in CFS there is reduced blood flow in the brain stem. The same test used on those without CFS but with depression did not find the same pattern. The brain stem is important because it controls the heart rate, blood pressure, swallowing, coughing, breathing and unconsciousness. Reduced blood flow seriously affects brain function; the energy requirements for the brain are far higher than for any other part of the body.

The cerebrum, which is divided into two hemi-spheres, is essential to thought, memory, consciousness and the higher mental processes. The thalamus, part of the midbrain, acts as a transmitter between the spinal cord and the cerebral hemispheres. Within the thalamus is the limbic system, which is concerned with memory, learning and the emotions. Beneath the thalamus is the hypothalamus. Research has shown that CFS patients have significant memory deficits, far worse than implied by the set of criteria used by the American Centers for Disease Control. This pattern is consistent with temporal-limbic dysfunction and significantly different from depressed and normal control subjects.

Hormones and the endocrine system

Hormones are chemical messengers which travel via the bloodstream. They regulate automatic responses, and bring together bodily functions. As such they form part of our endocrine system. The endocrine system, which works in close cooperation with the nervous system, keeps us 'in tune' with ourselves and our environment.

Hormones are also manufactured in glandular tissue found in organs such as the intestines and lungs. Mostly, the function of hormones is to control the trillions of cells which make up the body. Thus, for example, the function of the thyroid hormone is to determine the rate at which cells use up food substances and release energy. Neurotransmitters also act as hormones and vice versa.

The role of the hypothalamus

The hypothalamus is found in the base of the brain, and has connections with the midbrain. It is a link between the nervous system and the endocrine glands. One of its major functions is to relay impulses and stimuli between the brain and organs such as the kidneys. The hypothalamus is concerned with such vital functions as eating, sleeping and temperature control – all of which are affected by CFS.

Many PWCs develop food intolerances and digestive problems. Irritable bowel syndrome, with nausea, gassiness and bloating, diarrhoea, abdominal cramps and constipation, is often diagnosed before a later diagnosis of CFS. Sleep problems include difficulty falling asleep, early waking or frequent wakings in the night. The problem is that increasing activity to enhance sleep can also lead to a relapse, but total bed rest is not recommended, either.

PWCs become extremely sensitive to heat and/or cold, and some regulate heat loss by wearing hats indoors. Some PWCs report low-grade fevers with night sweats, especially in the upper part of the body. If you shake the hand of a PWC on a summer day, you may recoil at the freezing sensation when you touch them. Whichever extreme is present, hot or cold, the thermostat seems to be faulty, and this may originate in the hypothalamus.

The pituitary

The pituitary is located in the base of the brain, and is connected to the hypothalamus. They work together to control many aspects of the body's metabolism (its life-maintaining processes). The pituitary not only produces its own hormones, but it also affects the hormonal production of the other glands.

Two pituitary hormones which have been shown to be imbalanced in CFS are prolactin (excess) and growth hormone (deficient). Eighty per cent of growth hormone is produced during delta-stage sleep (the deepest period of sleep), which is often lacking in CFS, and it has a direct effect on the repair and regeneration of muscles – muscle pain and involuntary twitching are often found in CFS.

The thyroid

The thyroid gland is found in the neck, just below the level of the larynx. The thyroid hormone is thyroxine, whose overall effect is to control the amount of energy that the cell uses and the amount of protein that it manufactures; it is essential for life.

The adrenals

The adrenal glands are found just above the kidneys. Adrenalin and noradrenalin – known as the 'flight and fight' hormones because they are used by the body to prepare for danger and stress – are secreted from the centre of the gland. It is not surprising that the adrenals are closely linked to the nervous system. When signals are given to increase the production of adrenalin, blood and energy are reduced in non-essential functions, such as digestion, and diverted to the heart and the muscles.

Nowadays much of our 'alertness' to danger is not the result of physical threat but of emotional pressure, particularly stress which we feel is beyond our control. Problems in adrenalin production arise when these' dangers' place the body constantly on the alert.

Almost all of us feel the effects of lowered adrenal functioning at some time in our lives, usually following a bacterial or viral infection, or after mental or emotional stress. As well as those stress demands which are constant, adrenal insufficiency and adrenal exhaustion are encouraged by dietary deficiencies. When our adrenals cannot keep up we resort to stimulants – tea, coffee, cigarettes, alcohol, drugs – which further worsen the problem because they lead to adrenal exhaustion and the fatigue gets worse. Other symptoms of adrenal exhaustion are low blood pressure, poor circulation, cold or burning hands and feet, drowsiness during the day, wakefulness on lying down – hence insomnia – rapid and irregular heartbeat and brain fog.

One of adrenalin's functions is to reduce lactic acid levels. Lactic acid is produced by physical activity and shallow breathing. Too much lactic acid leads to fatigue, depression and lethargy, and PWCs have been shown to produce excess lactic acid.

The outer covering of the adrenals, the cortex, releases a series of hormones known as steroids, of which aldosterone, which controls water retention in the body, and cortisone, are the most important. During periods of prolonged stress there is extra demand for cortisone and the pituitary secretes the hormone ACTH in order to stimulate its production. Increased demand for more cortisone, however, leads over time to reduced output. So the link between stress, the nervous system and the immune system is strong.

With some types of CFS it seems that there may be a failure in the proper activity and balance of the hypothalamus, pituitary and adrenal (HPA) axis, resulting in low cortisol production and adrenals which cannot respond to the demands made upon them. The most extensive research on how the HPA works in PWCs has been carried out at the American National Institute of Health, where it was shown that CFS patients have significant memory deficits. This pattern was consistent with temporal-limbic dysfunction and significantly different to depressed and normal control subjects.

Muscle function, energy metabolism and oxygen take-up

Nerve cells transmit messages to and from the muscles, and blood cells play a vital part in bringing oxygen to power this process. An essential component is ATP, the chemical catalyst that helps to produce energy in every living cell. Without oxygen ATP is only produced in small amounts, and there is a build-up of lactic acid which, as we have seen, causes fatigue. During heavy activity with little oxygen, muscles produce lactic acid, which further reduces energy and strength. This is felt in the muscle ache following strenuous exercise.

PWCs have been found to have an excess of lactic acid, even without excessive use of muscles. It is interesting to note that research has shown that PWCs use a far higher proportion of energy for what is called 'resting strength' – the energy needed merely to sit, digest and carry out normal bodily functions – than others.

Over half the energy of a healthy person is derived from the aerobic metabolism of fat, with the balance coming from carbohydrate and protein. Fat yields approximately twice as much energy per gram as carbohydrate or protein. Carbohydrates become a main source of energy only when exercise exhausts the limit of fat metabolism, during anaerobic exertion. They are primarily stored in muscle tissue and the liver in the form of glycogen, in very limited quantities compared with fat.

Tests reveal that many PWCs use anaerobic energy within a couple of minutes of light walking, and specific metabolism tests reveal that many of them obtain 80 per cent of their energy from carbohydrate when resting. Research indicates that those with CFS have shifted towards inefficient anaerobic metabolism, and that sitting and slow walking in CFS is equivalent to a healthy person's running and sprinting.

Linked to this, experiments have shown that many PWCs have reduced oxygen uptake, which is a measure of aerobic fitness, or how efficiently the body utilizes oxygen. This reduced uptake is equivalent to that of someone with emphysema or a 70-year-old with a heart condition. It is thought to be linked to a mitochondrial dysfunction whereby the key chemical that helps to transport fat across the cell membrane, to be turned into energy, fails to function.

Efficient electrical impulses depend on the right balance of sodium and potassium ions – electrically charged metal molecules – inside and outside the cell membranes. Without the correct balance membranes may find it harder to conduct an electrical impulse, leading to fatigue. The levels of potassium in the blood rises during exercise, when it is released from the muscles, and later falls as it is redistributed throughout the body. Potassium works with sodium to maintain the nerve system's ability to send messages and is therefore essential to nerve and muscle function. Very low levels caused by diarrhoea and vomiting can cause muscle paralysis.

Australian research at the Royal Adelaide Hospital, reported in the Medical Journal of Australia, found that PWCs had a significantly lower total body potassium than matched controls. Potassium release from muscles into the bloodstream was significantly delayed in PWCs. The researchers suggest that this may contribute to fatigue in CFS. Potassium works with sodium to maintain the nerve system's ability to send messages and is therefore essential to nerve and muscle function.

Breathing

At rest an adult should ideally breathe lightly, superficially and only through the nose. Most people think they breathe shallowly but in fact they breathe very deeply. In response to stress, both physical and emotional, the heart rate increases and we breathe more deeply. When we overbreathe, or hyperventilate, we loose valuable carbon dioxide. Since carbon dioxide regulates the departure of oxygen from the blood, a fall in carbon dioxide results in reduced oxygenation of tissue and vital organs. This in turn affects the immune and nervous systems. A vicious cycle therefore sets in because the breathing centre in the brain is affected, causing a further increase in breathing rate and an even greater loss of carbon dioxide. Carbon dioxide deficiency can cause irritability, sleeplessness, stress problems, unfounded anxiety and poor digestion.

Hyperventilation is sometimes a significant perpetuating factor in CFS, and many of the symptoms found in carbon dioxide deficiency are also found in CFS. A number of doctors and practitioners try to help CFS by treating hyperventilation through correcting bad breathing patterns.

Bringing it all together: the persistent viral hypothesis linked to chemical toxicity

It is interesting that muscle weakness in polio survivors is profoundly increased when it is cold, so much so that at 20°C the nerves conduct as if they were at 13 degrees. Dr Richard Bruno, a clinical psychophysiologist, links this with a damaged autonomic nervous system and hypothalamus, caused by viral damage in the brain. The symptoms experienced by polio survivors in post-polio syndrome and CFS are the same, suggesting the possibility, according to Dr Bruno, that they share the same disease process, as evidenced in similar brain areas affected in brain scans.

Neuroscientists agree that subtle disruptions of brain chemistry, particularly in the hypothalamus, are intimately involved in CFS. They suspect that it may be caused by a persistent virus, but possibly also by chemicals which are toxic to the brain. Viruses which have been implicated in neuronal disruption are thought to evade detection by the body's immune system, using chemical tricks to confuse and disrupt virus detectors in the cell.

Although the last word is still some way off, for the time being it may be useful to think in terms of different causes working together at once, or one after the other. Abnormal permeability of the blood/brain barrier, as with MS, allows toxic chemicals or viruses access to sensitive brain cells. Indeed, the damage to brain cell membranes may have been caused in the first place by chemicals which do not form a normal part of the body. The immune system then becomes dysfunctional, so that it is more difficult to eliminate viral activity. Some people may have allergic reactions to pollutants, and in others their ability to detoxify them may have been overwhelmed. For the body, the consequences are as described above.

Clearly, this is only one hypothesis amongst many. However, it does seem to be a useful way to connect the research already completed, with the preliminary results of research which is still in progress. In other sub-groups of CFS – and it is important to bear in mind that there may be several – it may well be that psychological factors predominate, but this does not preclude the other causes from co-existing, or from applying elsewhere. The next few years will hopefully tie up all these ends, and bring even more understanding to this complex illness than is available now. For now, however, rather than try to understand this chapter immediately, focus more on the next chapters. They suggest positive ways to deal with the symptoms and the overall condition.

CHAPTER 3

Causes and risk factors

At first those researchers who felt that there was more to CFS than psychological causes concentrated their efforts on hunting for a virus. Now many admit that although it acts like a viral illness in that it comes and goes, with numerous symptoms, a virus may not be the only triggering factor. Indeed, the virus, or viruses, may only take hold because of other weakening effects on the body. Many researchers are now publishing findings which point to toxic damage from chemicals in our environment. We may also find that stress plays a significant part in undermining our defences to the extent that CFS takes hold.

Given that CFS is in all probability a multi-causal illness, the following have been suggested as possible contributing factors, in combinations that vary according to the individual and his or her particular history:

- heredity
- viral infection
- chemical exposure and toxicity
- lifestyle – emotional stress and how we nourish ourselves
- immunizations
- allergies and food intolerance
- overuse of antibiotics
- amalgam fillings
- chronic undiagnosed infection
- geopathic stress and low-level radiation

- trauma such as surgery, accidents or stressful life events
- hyperventilation

Heredity

Our external features are determined by our inherited genes. So is our immune system, and this may be a factor in CFS. Certainly, in homoeopathic medicine our constitution is as important as the specific symptoms, and genetic studies have demonstrated common weaknesses in patients with CFS. This does not mean that there is nothing to be done to avoid becoming ill or getting better; there are many other factors which contribute to wellness which are under our control.

Viral infection

Viruses are suspected because of the historical links of CFS with polio epidemics, and because the illness usually starts with an infection (which will often be considered trivial at the time). The existence of areas with an unusually high incidence of CFS, such as southwest Scotland, suggests that infection may play a part. But although it may trigger an outbreak so that some people develop CFS, that does not mean that CFS itself is infectious.

There is evidence that enteroviruses (polio, Coxackie A and B, echo and other numbered strains) are capable of infecting a wide range of specialized cells and tissues. Enteroviruses are known to affect muscles and nerves in particular, and these are of course the two main tissues affected in CFS. The resultant disturbances also fit the symptoms of CFS. Other agents, especially Epstein Barr virus, influenza and chicken pox may also be activated in CFS. Enteroviruses are spread through the faeces of those infected, but many of us carry the virus with no ill effects. Somehow, the right conditions occur in CFS for it to become activated.

But if CFS were contagious than we would expect a large number of spouses to have contracted the disease. In fact, it is rare for this to happen, even after some time. Thus Dr Charles Lapp, of Charlotte, USA, in a review of his practice, found the incidence of spouse/spouse illness to be about 6 per 1,000, but even these couples fell ill at approximately the same time, which suggested that they were both exposed to something simultaneously.

Some viruses may produce a hidden infection that does not trigger the body to fight back. These 'hit and run' infections could cause long-lasting problems after the virus has disappeared.

Chemical exposure and toxicity

Toxicity can come from the air we breathe being polluted with heavy metals, pesticides and chemicals, from preservatives in food, from poisons in tobacco, drugs and alcohol, from water that is affected by heavy-metal contamination and from medical drugs. The American chemical industry alone produces and releases into the environment around 900lb of chemicals per year for every person in the country. Without good nutrition the body has an uphill struggle getting rid of toxins, and fatigue usually follows.

We should also remember that the body has to try to eliminate naturally occurring toxins called metabolic waste. To do so it needs good nutrition and exercise; our sedentary lifestyles do not encourage this.

Organophosphates

Anecdotal evidence suggests that exposure to synthetic chemicals, including solvents, organophosphates (OPs) and pyridine compounds, can play a role in causing some illnesses. Mark Purdy is a British organic dairy farmer and researcher into the effects of chemical use in farming. He argues that degenerative nervous disorders, including some forms of CFS, can be caused by OPs. He points out that many people who prove susceptible to CFS also carry the gene for Gilbert's disease, a condition in which the capacity of the liver to eliminate some types of OP and other chemicals may be impaired.

OPs get into humans largely through the food we eat. They can be present in milk and are sometimes used to protect grain reserves from weevil damage. They are also sometimes sprayed on fruits and vegetables to stop them going mouldy.

A number of cases of CFS have been reported amongst farm workers who have been exposed to OPs. In the Scottish islands of Lewis and Harris, where there are four times as many CFS cases as in the rest of Scotland, all of the 22 men and 40 women with CFS have worked with OPs in sheep dips or on fish farms. This possible link is being researched in a two-year study into OPs used in sheep dips and their effect on human ill health. Dr Sarah Myhill, a British doctor with a rural practice of 1,800, identifies two types of possible reaction to sheep dipping: those with clear evidence of neurological damage, as in Parkinson's disease, and the majority who have 'soft' neurological symptoms and signs, and the symptoms of CFS. She suggests that perhaps the present rise in CFS is due to increased individual susceptibility to low-dose chemical exposure.

One of the symptoms of CFS is chemical sensitivity – an inability to tolerate even normal domestic chemicals in washing powders, cleaning agents and perfume. Dr Myhill finds that her 'problem' patients are those with chemical sensitivity and/or overload. Soldiers suffering from Gulf War syndrome, who report similar symptoms to CFS, were exposed to multiple chemical cocktails, and she notes that they have the same pattern of abnormalities of neuro-endocrine function.

Lifestyle

Stress is a response the body makes to demands which are perceived as difficult or frustrating, and the response to this stress in the body is not always recognized. Stress is not only caused by external factors but is also generated internally by our hopes and aspirations, beliefs, attitudes and personality attributes. For example our expectations of ourselves can sometimes be unrealistic, leading to stress when we fail to measure up, or physical strain when we continue to push ourselves, despite the need for rest.

Hormonal by-products of stress include cortisol and prolactin. Cortisol subdues the immune system, of which the most susceptible part is the mucosal system, in particular the protective cover to our digestive tract. If the immune system is weakened over time by stress, this can further increase the load, and can result in CFS.

Some PWCs recognize that before their illness they were affected by stressful life events and reactions. For them, recovery needs to involve a new way of coping with stress. This is hard with CFS because of the body's inability to deal with stress once it has been pushed into chronic ill health. (See the chapters on self-help for positive suggestions for coping with stress.)

Apart from emotional stress, we also 'stress' our bodies when we fail to nourish ourselves with good food and good nutrition. This is a fundamental part of how we allow ourselves to become ill. Chapters 5 and 7 give guidelines on how to improve your diet.

Immunizations

Some PWCs report that their illness started after vaccination, or more than one vaccination given over a short period of time. Some experts suggest that the long-term effects of virus particles in the bloodstream from vaccinations could trigger CFS when the conditions are right. The recent media coverage of Gulf War syndrome, with the suggestion that it might have resulted from military personnel being subjected to numerous vaccinations together with chemical exposure, is interesting. It could throw new light on the role of immunization in health, when combined with other triggers. However, some of the doctors who focus primarily on the psychological factors in CFS, rather than the environmental, are also the ones who cast doubt on the existence of Gulf War syndrome. New research should help to settle this disagreement in the next few years.

Allergies and food intolerance

One of the symptoms of food intolerances can be fatigue. Many PWCs have a range of food intolerances, sometimes predating their CFS. These are sometimes slow to take effect, and therefore hard to pinpoint, and affect the body in ways similar to CFS. Obviously, if you can tackle intolerances by avoiding the foods which affect you, and heal the damaged gut lining which may be a contributing factor, you can lessen the burden of nutritional stress that may prevent recovery from CFS.

There are many theories about the rising incidence of food intolerances – the overuse of antibiotics, the decline in breast-feeding which affects immunity, the poorer quality of the food we eat, the almost universal acceptance of vaccinations and their effect on immunity, the increase in pollution and our toxic environment, and the effect of stress on digestion.

Many PWCs find that cutting out certain foods helps enormously. The common culprits are dairy products, wheat and yeast. A recent study in the *Lancet* suggests that gluten, which is found in wheat, rye, barley and oats, was not tolerated in three-fifths of the 53 patients with CFS who were tested. Some of the symptoms were alleviated when they cut these foods from their diet. Gluten sensitivity causes inflammation of the small bowel lining and neurological symptoms resulting from degeneration of the peripheral nerves and the spinal cord.

Overuse of antibiotics

There are two aspects to this problem: first, the overuse of antibiotics which occurs when we take them repeatedly, and secondly the exposure to antibiotics which we face when we eat meat which is intensively reared. Factory farming could not survive without antibiotics.

In the USA Dr Carol Jessop reported data from 1,000 patients with CFS at a conference held in 1989. Eighty per cent of the patients had had recurrent antibiotic treatment as a child, adolescent and adult for ear, nose and throat infections, acne or urinary tract infections. Furthermore, 60 per cent developed a sensitivity to many antibiotics over time. In killing harmful bacteria, antibiotics also wipe out beneficial bacteria, which in turn encourages fungal (candida) overgrowth to take hold. This leads to 'leaky gut', whereby the lining of the gut wall is damaged, possibly leading to viral access to other parts of the body.

Many people with CFS also suffer from candida overgrowth. Geoffrey Cannon, in his masterly book *Superbug: Nature's Revenge*, exposing the dangers of overuse of antibiotics, argues for more research on their possible role in serious chronic fatigue states. There are many anecdotal stories of PWCs recovering or nearing recovery when they follow treatment for candida overgrowth.

Amalgam fillings

Dental amalgam has been used to fill teeth since the early 1800s and used to be considered safe. However, studies now show that mercury vapour is continually released from amalgam fillings, and that dental amalgam is the major source of mercury exposure in the general population. The mercury vapour enters the blood via the lungs and mucous membranes in the mouth. It can penetrate cell membranes, and cross the blood/brain barrier. Some people may be sensitive to these minute amounts of mercury, which has been shown to affect the immune system and metabolism. Infections already present may be made worse. Some practitioners are convinced that their clients only responded to treatment for nutritional deficiencies and food intolerances in CFS when their mercury amalgam fillings were removed.

Chronic undiagnosed infections

Recent research demonstrates a higher than normal prevalence of local and general susceptibility to infections in CFS. Evidence was found for a reduced or unstable immune control or delayed immune reaction to persisting viruses or bacteria. Common infections or environmental factors are some of the possible triggers which are suggested by this research.

Some practitioners agree, on the basis of patient histories, that chronic undiagnosed infections can be part of the overload which leads to CFS, apart from resulting from it. Common problems arise from candida overgrowth in the gut (*see* chapter 7), chronic nail infections, *helicobacter pylori* which causes chronic indigestion and acidity, pelvic inflammatory disease (low-grade womb infections), prostatitis in men and chronic gut parasites. Persistent bacterial infections, for example in the teeth, tonsils or appendix, can sometimes remain undetected.

However, this aspect of CFS is still considered to be marginal or 'fringe'.

Geopathic stress and low-level radiation

Whilst we all accept the benefits of electricity, we often fail to appreciate its risks, apart from direct contact in the form of shocks. The Russians were the first to identify a possible risk when workers were found to have a higher incidence of illness when exposed to electric fields. Other research shows that 25 per cent higher rates of leukaemia are found in workers exposed to strong electromagnetic fields in the workplace. Scientists have found that mental performance could be impaired, stress induced and the immune system weakened as result of electromagnetic pollution.

Despite disagreement on the levels of danger, there is general agreement that, depending on the frequency, electric currents can contribute to both health and disease, affecting different functions of the body and the brain. Anecdotal evidence suggests that some PWCs are highly sensitive to electromagnetic fields, and a few react when close to overhead power lines. Others seem to react to levels of exposure far lower than those which would affect most people.

Some practitioners and scientists attempt to demonstrate that health can also be affected by geopathic stress. This refers to the harmful effects upon health from energy fields associated with a particular place, usually where we spend the most time, in the home or at work. These natural electromagnetic fields are created by under-ground running water, certain mineral concentrations, fault lines and underground cavities.

One expert in Britain, who went into the homes of 3,000 PWCs, noticed that the effects of geopathic stress were worse when combined with exposure to electro-magnetic fields from within the home, such as clock radios near the head, metal beds and bedsprings, electric blankets, radiators and transformers. This suggestion is considered by most doctors to be beyond serious consid-eration, however, and may, indeed, have no relevance. Nevertheless, if, after trying everything else, your prob-lem remains it may be worth while finding out more about this possible, but not proven, causal contribution. Changing to a wooden bed, sleeping in a room without electrical equipment plugged in, and using hot-water bottles instead of electric blankets could all help 'clean up' your environment, and lessen the load.

Trauma

The onset of CFS occurs abruptly in 75–90 per cent of cases. Although the most common trigger is a flu-like ill-ness, some people appear to be pushed over the edge by physically and/or emotionally traumatic events such as surgery, accident or injury. A combination of stressful incidents, such as bereavement, job loss or moving home, can also contribute to the overload which triggers CFS.

Hyperventilation

Most people tend, while at rest, to breathe too deeply. This may cause and perpetuate the symptoms of CFS. See the section on Breathing, pp23–4.

What this means for people with CFS

The causes listed above mostly stem from the environment, your lifestyle, your past medical history and your response to stress. The good news is that because of this emphasis there is much that you can do to help yourself. Beyond that, of course, there is the problem of finding help. The next chapter takes you through the early stages of CFS – the diagnosis, and what you are likely to be offered by conventional medicine.

CHAPTER 4

Conventional treatment and procedures

The official line

The accepted view in conventional medicine is that although the PWC may have had flu to start with, his or her problems have arisen because for a variety of reasons, usually considered to be psychological, the symptoms persist. In some of the medical literature in Britain patient support groups or the media are blamed for telling people what symptoms to expect – the implication is that the symptoms of CFS occur once the person finds out about them in the media.

There are some people who exhibit this form of behaviour, which doctors call somatization. These people may have difficulty in identifying their own feelings, and tend to experience bodily symptoms rather than anger, fear or sadness. Sometimes traumatic events are repressed, and the body maintains the tension patterns, thus producing symptoms and fatigue. They may fall ill and can be more susceptible to disease. Hyperventilation and depression can also result.

Patient support groups have been resistant to the somatization argument when it underpins CFS treatment such as exercise beyond the PWC's limits, or full-dose antidepressants, which usually cannot be tolerated. The problem of communication between doctors who take the somatization view, and patients who seek confirmation of their symptoms as 'real', can lead to tension and feelings of being misunderstood. The need to be emotionally supported or 'well held' is vital for those with CFS, a point which is emphasized in *Chronic Fatigue Syndrome: Information for Physicians* published by the National Institute of Allergy and Infectious Diseases in September 1996 in America.

Depression and CFS

Depression does not seem to be the cause of CFS, although it shares several of its characteristics and may follow from having it. The symptoms below are those which are found in both depression and CFS.

- fatigue
- agitation and restlessness
- sleeplessness or excessive sleeping
- weight changes
- impaired concentration
- lethargy
- decreased libido
- lowered activity level
- loss of interest or enjoyment in life

But the fact that these symptoms are shared should not hide the significant differences between the two conditions. These are:

- Most CFS starts suddenly with a flu-like illness. This is not the case with depression, which usually comes on gradually. When depression is sudden it is part of a bipolar (manic) disorder not found in CFS.
- The majority of PWCs do not have a history of major depression.
- Whereas local outbreaks of CFS are common, and it has been known to occur in epidemic form, this cannot

be said of depression, which is very much an individually occurring problem.

- Symptoms characteristic of depression, such as suicidal tendencies, guilt, pessimism and a sense of failure are not routinely exhibited in PWCs.
- Whereas most depressives do not want to be active, most PWCs do, but are physically unable to be so.
- for PWCs, exercising is particularly difficult and tiring, and can lead to relapse, whereas exercise usually makes depressed people feel better.
- CFS tends to persist for many years even when treated, which is not usually the case with depression. Treating CFS with full-dose antidepressants sometimes causes a worsening of symptoms, although low-dose antidepressants seem to help sleep problems at night.
- The immune abnormalities and cognitive dysfunction found in CFS are not found in depression.
- Research on reduced blood flow to the brain shows that different areas of the brain are affected in CFS from those affected in depression.
- PWCs often have a low tolerance of alcohol, which is not found in depression.

With CFS it is important to acknowledge the possibility that depression or anxiety could develop because of the experience of having an illness which is so debilitating, and the cause and treatment of which is not known. The possible consequences, such as loss of job, partner and career or negative experiences with health professionals also contribute to the possibility of reactive psychological problems.

The Royal Colleges Report on CFS (1996) concluded that the group which has more symptoms, profounder fatigueability, greater disability and a longer duration of the illness has the greatest association with psychological disorder. It judged the evidence to be weak for endocrine or immune function disturbances, as well as for structural or functional abnormalities of the brain or muscle. However, the report has been criticized on both sides of the Atlantic for incompletely examining the evidence, and for being selective in the research it chooses to 'prove' its preference for psychological causation. Chapter 2 gives other research findings which show a different pattern. Despite these differences between experts about its causes, there are a growing number of conventional doctors who are open to a multi-causal model of CFS.

The difficulties of diagnosis

We automatically assume that if our health breaks down someone else, who is trained in medicine or the healing arts, can put it right. The problem with CFS is that things are not so simple. There is no clear-cut route to diagnosis and acceptance, and the response varies from doctor to doctor – some do not even suggest any treatment. It may take you some time to confront your situation, and even longer before you finally get a diagnosis. And whatever expert you find to help you, you will have to work in partnership, and make judgments about the usefulness of that person's approach for you. You will also have to learn how to help yourself.

When you do decide to find out what this array of symptoms means, you may be discouraged by the lack of information – or the conflicting information – that is available. Your doctor will not have had any training about this syndrome as a student, because it has only recently been recognized. And even those doctors who know about CFS, are unlikely to have had time to read the latest research.

Despite these problems you must get a diagnosis, in order to rule out other possible explanations for your symptoms. One study in Dundee found that one-third of patients who had been diagnosed by their doctor as having CFS, were found in fact to have other medical conditions when extensive clinical and laboratory investigations were carried out. See Chapter 1 for a list of other illnesses which need to be ruled out.

Diagnosis

There is at present no one specific test for CFS – the usual tests show 'normal' results. Doctors who rely on tests more than the reporting of symptoms will find it hard to conclude that there is something physically wrong.

There is some controversy about how soon a diagnosis of CFS can be given. It is routinely recommended that a diagnosis before the person has had the illness six months is too hasty. On the other hand, leaving it this late risks long-term damage because sufferers are not educated about how to manage the illness through pacing. It is now recommended that CFS in children should be diagnosed after three months, rather than waiting six.

You may be given the following tests:

- haematological tests; full blood count
- thyroid function tests
- immunological tests
- checks for evidence of primary depression
- checks for presence of anxiety disorders
- investigation for hyperventilation syndrome
- further tests of any of the pathological causes of fatigue likely after history and examination

Dr Paul Cheney, one of the pioneering doctors in the USA to treat this condition, recommends three simple balance-function tests of central nervous system irregularity, known as the Romberg, tandem stance and augmented tandem stance tests. The Romberg test is the easiest to perform, followed by the tandem stance and then the augmented tandem stance.

The Collaborative Pain Research Unit, a joint team from Sydney and Newcastle Universities and John Hunter Hospital, Australia, argue that if CFS is more than somatization it should cause changes in the body's chemistry, which will be detectable in urine. Using a machine for detecting illicit drug use in athletes, they compared healthy controls with those with CFS. Decidedly different patterns emerged. The researchers asked patients to fill out a detailed survey of their symptoms, and this was then compared with their particular urine markers. They found that the patients fell into distinct groups, confirming that CFS was not one disease, but possibly as many as eight. Three of these groups accounted for two-thirds of the patients. It also seemed that the greater the overlap, the wider the range of symptoms; people with high amounts of the main markers were the sickest.

Many CFS patients in this study had a urine marker similar to compounds which block the production of energy in cells. There is evidence that it also stimulates pain centres in the brain. In addition some people with CFS seemed to have higher than usual pesticide levels in their bodies. This team is hoping to develop a simple dipstick test which could be done in the doctor's surgery and would tell patients which sub-group they belong to. So although there is still no cure, such a test would help patients discover what kind of CFS they have and so help them to manage their symptoms.

Dr Ian James, Consultant and Reader in Clinical Pharmacology at London's Royal Free Hospital

School of Medicine, thinks he has found not only a breakthrough in testing procedure, but also a way of alleviating symptoms. Following up doctors' observations that people with CFS have an abnormal pupil response when subjected to changes in light or focus, he found that pupil fluctuation was peculiar to PWCs. He suggests that it is caused by some kind of interference in the transfer of impulses from the brain to the eye. This means a deficiency of serotonin, whose job it is to pass impulses from nerves to cells. He has found that correcting the imbalance of serotonin can reduce some symptoms of CFS in some cases.

A survey of PWCs

A survey by the British charity Action for ME of 1,000 of its members gave the following results. It is worrying that despite being too ill to work, 67 per cent had no advice on management from their doctor.

Does your doctor accept that CFS exists?
Yes: 89%
No: 11%

Has your doctor given you advice on the management of the illness?
Yes: 33%
No: 67%

Have you had to stop working because of the illness?
Yes: 94%
No: 6%

Have you found benefit from any form of alternative therapy?
Yes: 62%
No: 37%

Treatment

No one therapy has been shown to be universally effective for CFS. The ones discussed here are those which have been tested or tried by doctors; those who have developed a more holistic approach are not included.

Conventional medicine likes to put new treatments through tests, usually double-blind placebo-controlled trials. This is a test in which two groups of patients are offered treatment, but only one group actually receives it. No one involved in the test knows who is receiving which 'treatment', so as to rule out the placebo effect – an improvement in a patient's condition which is due solely to psychological power and the expectations of the treatment.

In CFS relatively few treatments have been subjected to double-blind placebo-controlled trials because of the relapsing–remitting course of the illness over several years. There is also a difference between improvement in function and total cure. Of those treatments that have been rigorously tested, only four have been found to be superior to placebo. They are not widely used, however, because their effects have not been repeated in further trials. They are:

● the antiviral and immunoregulatory agent ampligen
● high-dose intravenous immunoglobulin
● intramuscular magnesium sulphate
● evening primrose oil

Other interventions that have been assessed so far include:

● antidepressants
● graded exercise programmes
● cognitive behavioural therapy

Some doctors also recommend relaxation and meditation, and psychotherapy and counselling, and these will be discussed in later chapters.

Far more emphasis has been placed on immunotherapy in the USA than in the UK, but the results of trials of this kind of therapy have been either disappointing or inconclusive. The two that have been most used are ampligen and immunoglobulin.

Ampligen

Ampligen has been tested and used in trials for some years. It works on the immune system and has been found to produce significant physical and cognitive improvements. However, important questions remain about the long-term use of the drug, and the higher the dose the greater the side effects. At the moment it is unavailable in the USA and the UK.

Anecdotal reports after trials ended in the USA found that many people felt the loss of their intellectual clarity and physical strength within a few days of coming off ampligen. By the third and fourth week some were back in wheelchairs, and after one trial nearly everyone became housebound again.

High-dose intravenous immunoglobulin

Immunoglobulin (written Ig for short) is a blood product that contains antibodies, which attach themselves to foreign substances to defend the body against infection. IgG is one of several types of immunoglobins or antibodies which are produced in the lymph cells to fight infection, and immunoglobulin is used in CFS primarily when total IgG is low.

Although trials have produced conflicting results, some patients do well on this treatment. However, intravenous immunoglobulin is extremely costly, and has side effects.

Intramuscular magnesium sulphate

Magnesium is vital for normal cell function. The transmission of nerve impulses depends on the correct balance of calcium and magnesium across the cell membranes. Muscle contraction and relaxation also depend on magnesium. It is interesting to note that many features of magnesium deficiency are also found in CFS, and a controlled study by Dr David Dowson (*see* Survey of PWCs: p43) indicated that many PWCs are deficient in magnesium. Treatment with a course of six weekly injections of magnesium sulphate benefited 80 per cent of the CFS group, and their red cell magnesium levels were significantly raised at the end of the trial.

Essential fatty acids and evening primrose oil

Magnesium loss can occur when cell membranes are subjected to free-radical damage thought to be caused by a redistribution of electrons. Essential fatty acids (EFAs) protect against this. They also kill enveloped viruses by destroying their fatty coats, and protect the normal function of interferon, the body's own antiviral agent.

Professor P O Behan of the Institute of Neurological Sciences at Glasgow University carried out a placebo-controlled study over three months, giving PWCs Efamol Marine, a particular brand of EFA, which contained gamma linoleic acid (GLA) and fish oil. Eighty-five per cent were judged to have improved in terms of fatigue, muscle pain, dizziness, poor concentration and depression. Levels of EFAs in the blood returned to normal in the treated group.

Because of the low concentration of GLA in Evening Primrose Oil, the daily doseage is high (9 capsules), so GLA from more concentrated sources can be substituted.

Antidepressants

There is only one published report of a controlled trial of an antidepressant, Prozac. This study concluded that it had no beneficial effect on any symptoms of CFS, suggesting that the depression in CFS has a different cause from the type which Prozac usually helps.

Tricyclic antidepressants seem to be the most effective when used in a low dose. They can be of help in relieving muscle pain and normalizing disturbed patterns of sleep. A useful test for CFS is to administer full-dose antidepressants and assess the reaction.

A study in Oxford found that of 55 patients, 4 felt they had 'greatly improved' with antidepressants whereas 13 stated that they had been 'made worse'. If your sleep is affected by CFS you may find that low-dose antidepressants are a positive way of lessening fatigue.

Graded exercise programmes

Some doctors believe that a regular programme of gradually increasing the amount of aerobic exercise is beneficial. Because the physical problem is usually seen to be caused by disuse, it is assumed that this therapy will reverse that damage. However, exercise programmes are more likely to be harmful to someone who, in the first year of the illness, still shows obvious signs of infection (eg fever, tender lymph glands, nausea or sweating).

It may also depend on whether or not the muscles are affected. Where there are abnormalities in the mitochondria, the cells' 'power stations', there is likely to be a problem sustaining aerobic exercise. This may possibly be due to persistent viral infection in the muscle cells.

Exercise, carefully monitored, may be helpful to someone who has been ill for some time, and whose muscles are very weak from lack of use. Even so it should be very gradually increased and carefully monitored. Exercise bikes should be avoided because they are too strenuous; gentle activity such as walking is more sensible.

Cognitive behavioural therapy

One form of therapy which is increasingly being used in the UK is cognitive behavioural therapy (CBT). It differs from graded exercise in that it emphasizes an agreed programme of activity developed jointly by the patient and the therapist. Moreover, activity is the key word, not exercise.

One problem is that CBT depends on the views about CFS of the person delivering it. Thus some doctors who believe that PWCs are in their predicament because of a hectic lifestyle, excessive focusing on their symptoms and a belief that recovery is not possible, use CBT to change the patient's own view that the illness is a physical one.

Problems with CBT may develop if the therapist tries to encourage patients to ignore symptoms which are better treated in another way. As with any therapy, a lot depends on who is administering it. Certainly, many PWCs learn how to pace their energies using this systematic approach and benefit from the regular appointments and clear objectives, and as a result feel a lot better. CBT could be a useful adjunct to other therapies.

An alternative to cognitive behavioural therapy

Dr Darrel Ho-Yen, a consultant microbiologist in Scotland, achieves excellent results with his CFS patients by starting from the understanding that they are ill, having first excluded those without CFS but with clinically active psychiatric disorders. By reinforcing their belief in the physical nature of the illness, as opposed to challenging it by suggesting it is 'all in the mind', he is not denying the role of psychological factors. However, he sees considerable psychological pain being caused by the wasted energy involved in patients' feelings of anger and frustration. Instead he encourages them to try to learn about their illness, and how it affects them, and to stop looking for an instant cure but, instead, to ensure that they do not overdo activity or ignore the illness.

The confidence that comes from being believed leads to empowerment and some control over the illness. Energy levels increase, as does activity. But he does not recommend greater activity until the PWC feels 80 per cent normal for over four weeks, so keeping a symptom diary is essential.

We will look more closely at the the interconnections between supportive care and self-help in the next chapter.

CHAPTER 5

Moving on to help yourself

The interesting thing about the majority of self-help techniques is that the same things that help physical problems often also help psychological ones. So gentle yoga breathing exercises will not only help to give your body more oxygen, but also make you feel mentally and emotionally stronger.

There is sometimes a time-lag between being advised what to do when you have an illness, and getting to the stage when you are ready to take that advice. This is the difference between acquiring and applying knowledge. This is particularly true with CFS, where there is brain overload, a great deal to learn, and not much energy to take in more than one thing at a time.

Despite the advantages of helping yourself, you need to work with someone else, preferably a doctor with a holistic perspective or a complementary therapist who has an understanding of nutrition and energy needs. This is because it is not easy to make the changes you will need in order to improve. There are bound to be set-backs, and many questions along the way. You will need reassurance that you are on the right track.

In general terms the self-help approaches work in three basic ways:

- by empowering you to take control
- by helping to rest your brain, not just your body
- by enhancing your coping patterns

Translated into actual procedures, self-help approaches take account of the need to:

- find out what is happening to your body
- keep records to chart ups and downs
- modify diet and improve nutrition (including cutting out food allergens)
- pace your activities with regular rest
- restore normal sleep patterns
- improve breathing
- learn relaxation techniques
- develop an exercise routine (gentle and within your energy limits)
- maintain a positive outlook
- care for your emotional and mental welfare

Some of these aspects will be dealt with in chapter 8.

Keeping informed

Understanding what is going wrong is vital as you start to assess what you need to do, both mentally and physically. One of the first things you will learn about CFS is not to expect an overnight cure. Resist the temptation to rush from one cure to another, especially if you have not tapped into your ability to help yourself.

Keeping a record to chart the ups and downs

If you are to develop new skills in pacing your energies you must build up an awareness of what brings on a relapse, and how symptoms fluctuate. Over time patterns may emerge. Dr Darrel Ho-Yen, who asks his patients to keep a diary, finds that it is lack of confidence which gets in the way of recovery. He allocates his patients energy scores on the basis of their entries. It is only when they have experienced a high enough score for some time that they can move on to extend their energy output.

Record keeping is not excessive focusing on symptoms. It is a major tool in your efforts to help yourself. It is of tremendous importance that you can see from day to day how what you are doing can influence the outcome. Although this comes under the heading of self-help, it is clear that it is more effective if you have someone monitoring your progress.

Diet and nutrition

Changing your diet and improving your nutrition are very much part of the self-help programme, although the use of food supplements requires help from professionals trained in nutrition. Food supplements are nutrients concentrated and put into capsules or tablets (although some, such as vitamin C, are also popular in powder form) and taken as a supplement to a normal diet.

Here are some tips for healthy eating and drinking:

- As far as possible buy organic food. You are aiming to cut down on the load of chemicals to which you are exposed. Meat and dairy products are laced with antibiotics, and organophosphates are found as residues in much of our chemicalized food.
- Scrub organic vegetables rather than peeling them. If you cannot get organic vegetables and fruit soak them in a dilute solution of apple cider vinegar or powdered vitamin C to remove some of the contamination from factory farming.
- Give your body sustainable energy by eating slow-releasing carbohydrates such as whole grains, pulses, vegetables and fruit. Aim to cut out sugar altogether.
- Drink plenty of clean, filtered water (up to 2 litres a day if you can) or herb teas rather than tea and coffee. Start the day with a mug of hot water and a slice of

lemon. This is a good way to detoxify the body after sleep and to encourage the bowels to work.

- Help your bowels by soaking some linseeds in apple juice or water overnight, and swallowing them with water before breakfast. They will become a bit like frogspawn, but try to crunch a few to benefit from the essential fatty acids they contain. Linseeds are the best way to achieve regular motions, especially as you cannot exercise very effectively. Alternatively, you can omit the soaking, grind them in a coffee grinder and sprinkle them on food. Always do this when they are fresh, and store any left-overs in a screw-top jar in the fridge, but only for a couple of days.

- Cut out alcoholic drinks. One of the effects of CFS on the body is to make you intolerant of alcohol. Your liver is not able to cope with it.

- You may find it difficult to eat raw foods, especially if you have a problem with candida overgrowth. This is because you need warming foods. Get into the habit of making sustaining soups which are quick and easy to do if you have a liquidizer. Freezing small quantities for the days you are feeling unwell is a good idea.

- Lessen the load by cutting out foods to which you are intolerant. Many PWCs have a problem with dairy products, which are mucous forming. If you are eating plenty of fresh green vegetables and seeds, you should be getting enough calcium, although you may need to supplement your intake. Substitute goat cheese for cow's milk cheese. Make porridge with water for a sustaining breakfast, although you may need to try cutting out wheat and other gluten-containing grains such as rye, oats and barley.

- Be careful not to cut too much out of your diet without learning about new foods which are better for you. The next chapter has advice on healing your gut wall, which could improve your tolerance of foods.

- To sustain energy you may need to eat little and often.
- You may find it easier to digest food if you follow the principles of food combining – not eating proteins and carbohydrates during the same meal. This theory suggests that where there is a mixture of both kinds of food, neither is properly digested, which may lead to energy depletion and poor absorption. There are many books available which introduce this way of eating (*see* Appendix B).

Pacing your activities with regular rest

It is true to say that everybody with this illness thinks that when they have energy they can use up what is in the bank, which leads them into 'overdraft'. In fact, 'save it' should be the motto. Knowing when to stop an activity is hard, but stopping well before you are tired is essential to avoid a relapse. The following energy ration card was devised by Martin Le Grice in his helpful little booklet *Managing ME*.

Energy ration card – (example only)

Exercise		walk	10 mins
	or	swim	4 mins
Mental work		writing/computer	1 hour
	or	reading	2 hours
Social interaction		phone	2 x15 mins
	or	lunch/party	1 hour
Domestic chores		shopping	20 mins
	or	cleaning	20 mins
	or	washing	2 loads
	or	cooking	30 mins

Restoring normal sleep patterns

There are several strategies you can follow to enhance sleep. You can develop various anti-stress methods, together with breathing techniques and exercises as appropriate, or take a calcium/magnesium supplement before bedtime (in a ratio of 2:1), or a protein snack. One gram of vitamin B3 (niacinamide) taken at bed time helps those who sleep readily but cannot return easily to sleep after waking during the night.

Improving breathing

Learning how to breath properly is an easy self-help method that can help any problem, particularly CFS (See the list of BHMA tapes in Appendix C). Correct breathing is breathing with the abdomen, or stomach, not the chest (*see* figure 2). We start off in life doing this correctly, but over time we respond to stress by breathing shallowly from the chest. This can cause tiredness and muscle tenderness in the neck, shoulder and chest are often caused by overbreathing.

A simple breathing exercise, which is used in the practice of yoga, is to take a short breath in, and to follow with a longer breath out. Always breathe through the nose. Do this daily for several minutes at a time, in both a sitting and a lying position.

Good posture also encourages proper breathing, but holding yourself correctly may be difficult in CFS if you are in pain and fatigued. One of the best ways to improve posture is the Alexander technique (*see* pp90–3).

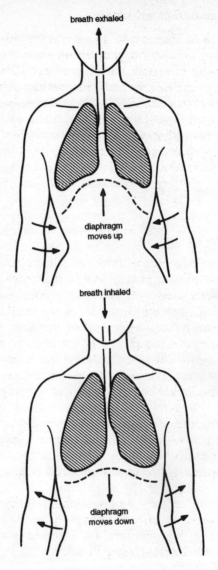

Fig. 2 Breathing correctly

Learning relaxation techniques

The need to be taught how to relax is an indication of how difficult it is to cut yourself off from the stresses and strains of everyday life. If you have CFS it is not good enough to relax the body without also relaxing the mind. This is because your brain is struggling to cope with overload. Learning to empty the mind, through practising relaxation, self-hypnosis or meditation techniques is a positive step. There are books, tapes, videos and classes so that you can find out which suits you. The pay-off may not be immediate, and you may need patience at first to keep practising.

Developing an exercise routine

Normal exercise programmes, which are competitive and geared to an outcome, and which involve perspiration and effort, are unsuitable for PWCs. But gentle exercise, which is within your energy limits, should be an important part of your daily routine. A useful exercise technique, which also works to calm the mind, is yoga, when given specifically for the needs of those with CFS. Yoga works not only physically on muscles and the skeleton but subtly on nerves, organs and glands.

Another useful approach comes from the Chinese art of chi kung exercises. This allows you to progress at your own pace, as with yoga.

See Appendix B for recommended reading in this field.

As with all activity, do not suddenly increase your level of exercise when you feel you have the energy to do so. Stay at the same level for a period of time, and only gradually increase it step by step.

Bonnie

Bonnie, 38, was first diagnosed with CFS when she was in her late twenties. She had been working very hard, and had caught a bug whilst working abroad, before which she had had a series of immunizations in close succession. At first she struggled to carry on working, despite her lack of energy and muscle pain. However, a complete relapse after exposure to paint fumes forced her to accept that struggling on was only making matters worse. Living on her own and bedridden, in desperation she asked a friend to look after her. He moved in to care for her for three months, during which time he helped her to sell her flat and find somewhere bigger, in order to have others to live with her more easily so that she would not be totally alone. Through very careful pacing of her energy and the use of co-counselling to help her reduce the stresses in her life, she slowly but surely improved. She also had help with candida control, and healing. The healing worked to give her energy boosts, which she 'topped up' every few months. Small walks to the shops were followed by longer ones to the park. She is now able to work part time, and continues her routine of yoga, co-counselling and a daily rest. She is not fully recovered, but she has made enormous improvements. Learning to pace herself was crucial.

Keeping a healthy mental and emotional outlook

Scientists now know that severe stress and strain can cause the immune system to weaken, allowing our defences to break down. Keeping a healthy mental and emotional outlook is vital, despite all the odds against achieving this when the illness is so poorly understood – it is not so poorly understood that nothing can be done.

Developing a healthy mental and emotional outlook depends on a realistic acceptance of the illness, before compliance with the need for fundamental changes in how you manage energy and how much you can achieve in any one day. Carrying on using old coping strategies, which may have involved mind over matter, may no longer be appropriate. Fighting CFS merely delays the necessary first stage of acceptance. This does not mean giving in to the illness. It means being honest about what is happening to your body and your mind, and then being able to work out strategies for recovery which are achievable.

The following is an extract from the American journal, the *CFIDS Chronicle*, Winter 1966. It is written by Dean Anderson, who describes himself as 'substantially recovered' after eight years of CFS.

> Over the years I read several reports by recovered or improving PWCs where they said they started improving after 'accepting' or 'resigning themselves' to their illness. Until recently I rejected this mind-set as defeatist or fatalistic. In America we are taught from early childhood that succeeding in life is important and that striving is the key to achievement.
>
> I initially viewed the healing process as one in which I would succeed through determination and hard work. I realize now that there is a problem with this type of thinking. It leads to a roller-coaster ride of emotional highs and lows. During the years that I consciously 'tried' to get well, I perceived remissions as steps up a ladder to recovery. The path would be ever upward. When relapses inevitably followed, I was devastated by apparent failure of my will and my conscious efforts. I believe today that a certain kind

of acceptance may be important to recovery. It is not a resignation to one's fate as a sick person. Rather, it is acceptance of the reality of illness and of the need to lead a different kind of life, perhaps for the rest of my life.

The 'effort' required to recovery from CFIDS is an exercise in discipline and hopefulness, not determination and striving. The discipline required is exactly the opposite of the discipline so valued in the scholar, professional or athlete. It is the discipline to recognize and adhere to one's known limitations and to follow a strict regimen without periodically lapsing. It is the discipline not to succumb to family or societal pressures to get back into the rat-race . . . What PWCs need to develop is the fortitude to accept their condition, even when others refuse to, and the discipline to do the things and adopt the hopeful attitude which will put them on the path to recovery.

CHAPTER 6

The natural therapies and chronic fatigue syndrome

In view of conventional medicine's inability to provide any really effective treatment, natural therapies have an especially important part to play in helping recovery from CFS. This chapter aims to introduce some of the 'gentle' alternatives. Do not be mislead by the term 'gentle'. In the right hands, these techniques can be very powerful and effective.

There is little that is new about most natural therapies. Many have been around for thousands of years. As the inadequacies of scientific medicine have become apparent over the last decade or so, these other traditional therapies have come to the fore. The list gets bigger all the time, so that finding your way through them can be confusing.

What is natural therapy?

There is some discussion, sometimes heated, about whether all natural therapies share one common idea or principle. Despite some unfounded claims that the natural therapies are not linked, the following principles apply across the board:

● There is no artificial separation between the mind and the body. Good health is a state of emotional, mental, spiritual and physical balance. Balance is fundamental to the basic notion of health in natural therapy. Disease comes from imbalance. This is found in the Chinese principle of yin and yang.

- There is a natural force in the universe. The Chinese call this *chi*, the Japanese *ki*, the Indians *prana*. In the West it used to be called by its Latin description *vis medicatrix naturae*, meaning 'natural healing force', which is shortened today to 'life force'. It is the role of different forms of therapy to tap into that and release its health-giving potential.

- Lifestyle, diet, inherited weaknesses and emotional extremes can all lead to imbalance. This view, expressed in different ways, is shared by all the natural therapies.

- As important as the above factors are, environmental and social conditions must not be ignored.

- Treating symptoms is not as effective for long-term recovery as treating the underlying cause.

- There is an emphasis on the importance of freeing the mind, and using it to develop positive thoughts rather than negative ones.

- Taking responsibility for your own health is essential. On the other hand, some of us may need to trust someone else, usually the therapist, to help us when we are stuck.

- In natural therapy, because we all have individual needs and physical weaknesses, no one treatment is the same. In addition, the therapeutic relationship between healer and patient is valued and encouraged in a way that modern medicine can only pay lip service to.

It is interesting that when scientific medicine has to respond to the success of some of the 'gentle' alternatives, it does so by saying that what they are good at is listening. It implies that that is the sum total of their success. Of course, most natural therapies place a high value on good listening in order to build up a thorough clinical picture and to establish trust and empathy. However, to restrict the value of natural therapies in this way seems to deny the other, equally valid, levels at which they work, such as directly on the body as in herbalism, or on the unconscious mind as in hypnotherapy.

Despite testimonies of the value of natural therapies from those who have successfully tried them, conventional medicine considers anecdotal evidence not scientific enough to be taken seriously. The natural therapies are more and more aware of the need to engage themselves in research as well as practice, but it may be some time before resources and energy are put into this important area. The experience with CFS, however, is that even when there is good research it may be neglected in favour of other research which is used, sometimes unfairly, to maintain the status quo.

Natural therapy practitioners build into their consultation time an opportunity to explain why changes are needed. This is in order to enlist the patient's cooperation. They understand that to be motivated, patients must know how the body works, and why changes are necessary in the way they live their lives. In this sense, therefore, it is easier for the natural therapies to be more holistic, because there is time to focus on the mind and the need for motivation for cooperation in treatment.

Therapies that are particularly helpful for CFS can be divided into three categories:

- physical therapies, which work obviously and directly on the body in a very physical way, both outside and in, such as chiropractic, herbalism, osteopathy, nutritional therapy and massage
- energy therapies, which are often based on Eastern

ideas of health and disease, focusing on balance and unblocking energy, such as acupuncture, homoeopathy and reflexology

- psychological therapies, which work positively for health on the mind and the emotions, such as meditation, psychotherapy, hypnotherapy, counselling, relaxation and biofeedback

These divisions are not rigid, however, and some therapies fall into more than one category. This is because they have a 'multilevel' effect, across the mind, the body and the spirit. Examples of this are yoga, massage and meditation.

Nutrition and diet, the core therapy for any recovery programme, is described in the next chapter. Herbalism, naturopathy, exercise and yoga are also important supporting therapies for everyone. Beyond these base-line therapies, the others can be selected to suit your needs.

CHAPTER 7

Treating the body

As we have seen, there is an overlap between the mind and the body, but there are some therapies which act mainly on the body and those are the ones we will be looking at in this chapter. Do not lose sight of the major factors for sustained recovery – support (both medical and personal) and rest for both the brain and the body, taken before the point at which you feel tired. If this core management approach is not in place in the early stages, all the other interventions will be undermined and have less chance to succeed.

Diet and Nutritional Therapy

What we eat has a direct effect on our body's ability to heal itself. However, changing the habits of a lifetime, is not easy, especially if your diet is based on convenience foods. Moreover, there is evidence that in CFS the body does not necessarily absorb and use all the nutrients you consume. You may need to take nutritional supplements under the guidance of a nutritional therapist to boost your intake.

Experienced practitioners do not recommend that nutritional supplements and herbs be used as single agents. You need a broad coverage of vitamins, minerals, essential amino acids and fatty acids before taking specific nutrient therapies for particular problems. No two PWCs are the same, so it is important not to try to treat yourself with nutritional supplements. The practitioner needs to monitor what is given, particularly as many PWCs tolerate nutrients poorly in the early stages of treatment. Gradually building up the number of supplements is to be recommended if there is a problem.

The main nutrients helpful in CFS are:

- vitamins
  - vitamin A (taken preferably as beta-carotene), an important antioxidant, 'mopping up' free radicals. Beta-carotene is found in all green and yellow fruit and vegetables, particularly apricots, alfalfa, beetroot and carrots.
  - the B vitamins. All B vitamins are important in protecting the body against disease and infection as well as being helpful in repairing tissue and bolstering against the effects of stress. B3 (niacin) and B6 (pyridoxine) are also important in helping EFAs work properly. B5 (pantothenic acid) is used in the body's response to stress, in the production of antibodies and in energy production. B vitamins are best taken as a complex (the whole range taken together). Sources in food are brewer's yeast, whole grains and meats such as liver and kidney.
  - vitamin C (ascorbic acid). This stimulates the immune system to make interferon, a natural antiviral agent. It is also antibiotic and antibacterial and helps the body use EFAs properly. Although it is present in most fresh, raw fruit and vegetables, the best sources are in citrus fruits, blackcurrants, rosehips and peppers.
  - vitamin E, the strongest of the antioxidants, which helps the muscles to use oxygen and is needed for the growth and repair of the skin. The richest natural sources are vegetable oils, fish oils, wheatgerm, leafy vegetables, egg yolk and legumes.

- minerals
  - magnesium, which is needed for nerve and muscle function, associated with calcium and vitamin C metabolism, with the normal working of the heart and with energy production, needed for protein, fat and carbohydrate synthesis. Food sources are soya beans, nuts, brown rice, fish, lentils, almonds and sunflower and sesame seeds.
  - calcium, the builder of bones and teeth, which is also involved with nerves and muscles, blood cholesterol levels and blood clotting, and in the function of the heart muscle. It is found in fish, nuts, root vegetables, eggs.
  - zinc, which is associated with growth and the immune system, is a potent antioxidant and part of important enzymes, and helps normal liver and brain function. Natural food sources are oysters, meat, pumpkin seeds, cheese and eggs.
  - potassium, with sodium, regulates the balance of water in the body and is needed in healthy muscle and nerve function and for energy-production enzymes. It also helps the intestinal tract. Natural food sources are dried fruit, nuts, raw vegetables.
  - selenium, an antioxidant which is an important component of enzymes. It works with vitamin E to protect the body against the ageing process. The richest natural sources are organic meats, fish, onions and garlic. Some areas have very low levels in the soil, however, so that supplementation is necessary.
  - iron, which transports oxygen in red blood cells and is needed for enzymes and the metabolism of B vitamins. It is found in shellfish, yeast, liver, dried fruit and wholegrain cereals.

- Other supplements
  - free-form amino acids, particularly taurine, an antioxidant. Amino acids are the building blocks of protein.
  - essential fatty acids. These can be obtained from evening primrose oil and gamma linoleic acid (GLA complex), and help maintain the cell wall.
  - CO Q 10. This is naturally present in the body, helps in the production of the chemical catalyst ATP, which is vital for energy production and enhances oxygen transportation. It takes up to a month to take effect.
  - herbal combinations for the support of the liver. They usually include some of the following: silymarin (milk thistle), turmeric, ginger root, goldenseal, artichoke and dandelion.
  - ginkgo biloba, which helps circulation to the brain and aids memory. It should be taken for at least six months.
  - bowel and gastric ecology formulations. They should be taken alongside, or before, support for the liver

The occasional use of intravenous nutrients for easier and more rapid absorption, is recommended by some CFS specialists in order to speed up recovery from viral infections and avoid the use of antibiotics. However, this intervention is frowned on by most doctors as unproven, costly and invasive.

Herbal medicine

Herbalism, the use of herbs and plants to heal, has been practised for thousands of years, and was the original form of medicine from which orthodox medicine, as we know it today, developed. Today some 85 per cent of the world's population rely on it for their major source of medication.

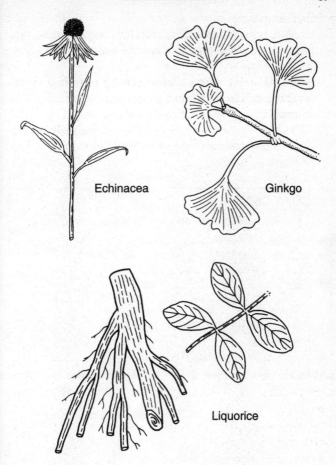

Echinacea

Ginkgo

Liquorice

Fig. 3 Herbs for CFS

Plant constituents are usually easily assimilated into the body without the adverse reactions or side effects associated with chemical drugs. Herbalists say that the reason the body reacts to drugs in this way is because the chemicals are too concentrated, without the benefits of the natural balancing effects of the whole plant. Herbalists also believe that when using the whole plant they are using more than the sum of the constituents. The vitality of the living plant is felt to be essential.

There have been few clinical trials involving herbal treatments for CFS, but many PWCs have benefited from their gentle but powerful effects. Ginkgo biloba has been shown by research to help improve circulation to the brain, and taken in 150mg capsules three times a day helps with dizziness.

Herbs for CFS

Some medical herbalists recommend the following herbs:

- anti-viral: echinacea
- immune support: echinacea, Siberian ginseng, panax ginseng, astragalus membranaceus
- liver stimulation and mild laxative: curled dock
- cleansing of the lymphatic system: cleavers, wild indigo, pokeroot
- liver support: dandelion root, barberry, black root, milk thistle, boldo
- adrenal support: borage, liquorice
- nervous system support: oats (as a tincture or simply as a porridge), lemon balm, betony, St John's wort, skullcap, vervain
- insomnia: wild lettuce, valerian, Jamaican dogwood, passion flower
- parasites: artemisia
- circulation to the brain: ginkgo biloba

Caution: Be wary of herbs which build up the immune system by giving more energy (such as Siberian ginseng). Energy levels should be increased slowly, so that you are not tempted to overdo things. You should avoid these problems by only consulting a qualified medical herbalist.

Naturopathy

Naturopathy is the umbrella term now used in most countries to cover a range of therapies. The term means natural treatment, and its practitioners are generally trained at specialist colleges in a range of skills that include acupuncture, herbalism, homoeopathy, osteopathy, massage, hydrotherapy, nutrition and diet.

There is a difference between modern naturopathy, which sees a role for nutritional supplements, and an earlier more idealistic approach which encouraged healing from the simple elements of fresh air, water, fresh food, fasting and exercise. The reality of our chemicalized environment and the effect of years of drug-based medicine, make this pure approach harder to sustain.

Naturopaths believe that infections only occur if the body departs from what nature intended for it. Becoming ill is natural, and getting better should follow the same natural principles. During treatment, symptoms can become worse before they get better. This is a sign that the body is fighting and eliminating poisons or toxins.

Sometimes naturopaths recommend a procedure called colonic irrigation for washing the gut clean and removing debris and mucus that may be interfering with the proper absorption of nutrients. Some PWCs have been helped by this procedure, but you should be careful to repopulate the gut with beneficial bacteria. They could be depleted unless more are reintroduced.

Hydrotherapy

Hydrotherapy is water therapy. Research has shown the benefit to some PWCs of cold baths, where the temperature is lowered gradually over a long period of time. Even if you are not brave enough to try them, you could benefit from the relaxing effect of neutral baths, in which the water temperature is the same as that of the body. This produces a relaxing effect on the nervous system. The head should be supported by a towel or sponge, and the water should be topped up periodically to the temperature of 97°F. The bath can last from 30 minutes to four hours, after which you should rest for an hour in bed.

Aromatherapy

This is one of the most popular complementary therapies, combining specific massage techniques with the whole spectrum of essential aromatic oils. Received over several weeks, aromatherapy can have deep and lasting effects. Some PWCs respond very well to this gentle approach and find it very helpful.

Osteopathy

Expert manipulation of the body, and especially the bones, muscles and tissues of the spine, has long been said to help a range of persistent and long-term (or chronic) problems. One manipulation technique is osteopathy, which means 'bone suffering'. It works to improve the overall structure of the body. Outside the USA, osteopaths are generally not doctors and train in special colleges, where there is more emphasis on naturopathic principles, all of which help CFS.

Some osteopaths suspect that one of the causes of CFS for some people could be problems in the upper back, which affect the sympathetic nervous system. As a result of treatment and the massage of soft tissue, blood supply to the brain should be increased and lymphatic drainage (the clearing of toxins from this vital part of the immune system) improved.

Chiropractic

Like osteopathy, chiropractic aims to restore balance by manipulation of the bones, muscles and tissues of the body, particularly the spine.

McTimoney chiropractic is a whole body manipulative technique which is particularly gentle.

Exercise and Yoga

Introducing some form of gentle exercise is essential for the recovery process, but it should be slow and sustained. Ideal forms are yoga and chi kung (*see* chapter 9), which are best combined with meditation or some other technique for resting the mind.

Using therapies to focus on symptom relief

The natural therapies work holistically by building up resistance and gradually removing obstacles to recovery. In this way they reverse the disease process. Symptoms are believed, unless psychological assessment suggests otherwise.

Leon Chaitow, a naturopath and osteopath, recommends treating the following problems in CFS:

- allergy and food intolerance
- bowel dysfunction
- yeast or viral activity
- anxiety
- hyperventilation
- muscle pain related to trigger points
- underactive thyroid
- adrenal stress
- sleep disturbance

Allergy and food intolerance

More and more nutritional doctors and nutritionists are coming to see that some of the problems of CFS are caused by many years of allergic responses to food and chemical sensitivities, compounded by stress. The pattern of allergies, leading to increased antibiotic use and slow recovery from viral infections, is usually present well before CFS takes hold.

With the help of a practitioner you should establish whether you have any foods which are causing problems, and any chemicals which you should eliminate from your environment. The Fibromyalgia Network in the USA did a survey (October 1993) to identify the foods which most commonly cause problems for people with fibromyalgia and CFS. They were identified as wheat and dairy products, sugar, caffeine, artificial sweeteners, alcohol and chocolate.

Elimination and rotation diets

There are no perfect laboratory tests for the diagnosis of food intolerances, but the main ones used are:

- blood testing
- electrical testing – vega testing
- muscle testing or applied kinesiology (AK)
- pulse testing

Food allergies and intolerances can be helped by eliminating the allergen through an elimination diet, with suspected foods being reintroduced to assess their effect. Or you may adopt a rotation diet, whereby the suspected foods are eaten once over a period of four days.

Bowel problems should be treated at the same time as, or before, allergies or intolerances, because yeast overgrowth or candida could be interfering with food absorption. Incomplete digestion because of low hydrochloric acid levels or poor digestive enzyme production can also lead to problems of food intolerance.

Bowel problems

Many seemingly unrelated symptoms are reduced or eliminated when the focus of treatment is on the bowel. The ecology of the gut is crucial to our health. Its lining is an important part of our defence against disease.

Your practitioner should be working with you to normalize the time it takes for waste to be eliminated; bowel transit time should range from 8 to 14 hours. You should have two or three effortless, odourless bowel movements a day. The use of nutrients and herbs can help to normalize bowel function – vitamin C, magnesium, probiotics (*see* p76), and specific herbal combinations.

Yeast or viral activity

Some studies point to the high percentage of PWCs who have problems of candida overgrowth, with a history of recurrent antibiotic use. Within the CFS support group literature there is much anecdotal evidence for the role of candida in CFS, either as a trigger or as an outcome. Nevertheless, you should be aware that many doctors remain unconvinced by the candida theory.

According to the yeast overgrowth theory, if beneficial bacteria are reduced significantly by antibiotics, a poor diet or stress, candida can overgrow and numerous symptoms can result. These are not necessarily confined to the digestive tract – for example, some PWCs have problems with thrush, cystitis, anal itching, bloating and wind and fatigue for many years preceding CFS. In this case it is thought possible that viruses can then overwhelm an already weakened immune system, gaining access to the body via a compromised gut (one which has been damaged by the roots of fungal organisms). Other PWCs may develop problems with yeast overgrowth later, once the viral trigger succeeds, because of immune dysfunction and poor digestion.

Candida albicans is the main yeast involved, and is

known best for its role in causing thrush. Helped by a high sugar diet, poor digestion and stress, it can change into a fungus, damaging the lining of the intestinal tract. This allows harmful toxins access to the bloodstream. Food intolerances can result, together with many of the symptoms found in CFS – extreme fatigue, irritable bowel, muscle and joint pain, sore throat, feeling 'spaced out', and intolerance of alcohol. Symptoms which are highly suggestive of candida overgrowth, although not always present, are a bloated stomach, anal itching, wind and sugar craving.

Probiotics

According to naturopaths the environment of the bowel is always injured in chronic illness, and probiotics are often helpful in CFS. The term is used to emphasize the positive role that the friendly bacteria play. Bacteria are living organisms capable of carrying out an enormous number of reactions which affect the body. They form a significant part of our bowel ecology: 30 per cent by weight of human faecal material is composed of bacteria. The two most numerous and most beneficial are *Lactobacilli acidophilus* and *Bifidobacteria*.

Probiotics:
- help to maintain the acidic pH in the large intestine, which in turn helps to control disease-causing organisms, including the fungal form of candida
- deprive other less favourable organisms of oxygen, food and iron
- help to digest lactose in milk
- are thought to lower blood cholesterol
- regulate immunity
- synthesize certain vitamins, and help the absorption of certain minerals
- are capable of producing certain antibiotic products

Weeding out candida is not to be recommended if you do not at the same time 'seed' the gut with probiotics, and 'feed' it with growth factors to encourage normal bowel bacteria, and nutrients to heal the gut wall. Because of the complexity of the problem, you should always work with a knowledgeable practitioner.

The order of treatment for restoring gut ecology varies between practitioners, but will usually include the following:

- Herbal and enzyme support for the liver is usually advised at the start of treatment. This is because the liver is often weak in CFS, and candida treatment increases the load.
- Some practitioners also start treatment with probiotic formulations of 20 billion microbes per day for a week or two, followed by 4 billion microbes per day, and natural antifungals (*see below*).
- Others start with a herbal combination product such as Eradicidin Forte, which contains artemisia annua, berberis and grapefruit seed extract. It has antiviral, antifungal and antibacterial effects.
- At some point your practitioner might introduce products to heal the gut wall. Those which combine NAG (N acetyl D glucosamine) and L-glutamine are the best. NAG is an active growth promoter of *bifidobacteria*, and aids the building of the connective tissues lining the intestinal tract. L-glutamine aids intestinal growth of the mucous lining the gut wall. Butyric acid is also useful, and is naturally found in butter.
- Other natural antifungals, are Candicidin, which has the most thorough action, a time-released caprylic acid formulation or a product derived from grapefruit seed extract. Candicidin works against many strains of candida, and is based on extracts of essential oils which are capable of acting beyond the gut wall. Caprylic

acid is a short-chain fatty acid found in human breast milk and coconuts.

● Garlic concentrate, or fresh raw garlic, is another natural antifungal. It is also antibacterial and antiviral. If you do not want to take fresh raw garlic, you should choose a product which retains the natural allicin content through freeze drying.

This kind of management should lead to slow and sustained improvement over weeks and months, as long as you follow a diet at the same time which cuts out sugar, refined carbohydrates and some fermented foods.

Some doctors still use antifungal drugs, such as Nystatin and Diflucan, but these should not be used without first trying the new and effective natural antifungals. Naturopaths say there is a danger, particularly with Nystatin, that long-term use merely destroys a limited number of strains of candida, allowing other resistant strains to remain unchecked. Treatment solely on the basis of antifungal drugs and diet, without attention to repopulation with beneficial bacteria and healing the gut wall is likely to fail.

Another problem is parasitic infestation, which is likely when the balance of bowel micro-organisms has been upset. Intestinal parasites coexist with their human hosts, but they are kept under control in a healthy person by the high level of acidity in the stomach. There are several natural antiparasitic herbs which can be used, of which the Chinese herb artemisia is the most effective.

Anxiety and hyperventilation
For many PWCs, their anxiety is a result of their symptoms, but it can also act as an aggravating factor, and your practitioner should take time to alleviate it. For example, breathing irregularities can cause anxiety states. Hyperventilation, or overbreathing, can be

reversed by learning to relax the muscles, practise correct breathing, and to achieve mental calm.

Leon Chaitow recommends a neutral bath for inducing deep relaxation and sleep enhancement (*see* 'Hydrotherapy' above).

Muscle pain related to trigger points

PWCs describe various types of pain in their joints, muscles, lymph nodes (especially those in their neck and armpits) and throat. No evidence has been produced to show that the muscular aches and pains of CFS have much to do with inflammation. But painful trigger points in muscles can arise, and they can be relieved.

Trigger points are highly sensitive points lying within tight bands of muscle which are painful when pressed. Pain or other symptoms are felt elsewhere in the body as a result of pressure on the trigger points, and using these muscles often results in pain. Trigger points are thought to be areas of increased energy consumption and lowered oxygen supply due to poor local circulation. The muscles in which trigger points are found are not able to reach their normal resting length, and are therefore held in a constant shortened position.

Trigger points become a self-perpetuating cycle and will not go away unless adequately treated. They are maintained and/or made worse as a result of repetitive and continuous musculoskeletal, emotional or other forms of stress.

It is thought that there is inadequate oxygenation and retention of acid wastes in overused muscles because of overbreathing, and these become painful and stiff. The muscles most affected in this way are mainly those of the neck, shoulder and chest. As a result they are constantly using energy in a non-productive way even during sleep. Incorrect breathing also restricts the spinal

joints which attach to the ribs, causing stiffness and dis-
comfort. The pain can be alleviated and minimized by:

- specific strain/counterstrain techniques, as in
  osteopathy
- rubbing the affected area
- acupuncture
- postural and breathing re-education

Underactive thyroid and adrenal stress

An underactive thyroid and poor temperature control,
leading to cold extremities, may be caused by a problem
with the adrenal gland. You may be asked to record
your temperature over three days. If it is more than half
a degree lower on average, some naturopaths may prescribe small doses of thyroid extract. There should be
extremely careful monitoring of body temperature and
pulse rate whilst using this approach.

Other hormonal systems are also affected in CFS. It is
now possible to have a test which charts the highs and
lows of adrenal function, on the basis of saliva samples
at different times of day. Treatment using specific nutrients can then be accurately targeted in an attempt to
normalize adrenal function.

Sleep disturbance

Apart from the use of various natural therapies you may
find relief from devices which use an electromagnetic
signal transmitted through a kind of microcomputer
worn round the neck or wrist. Powered by a tiny battery
or microchip, the signals are picked up by the nervous
system and passed to the brain. These signals 'fill in' the
missing frequencies found in CFS and are thought to
help sleep, energy levels and 'foggy brain'. Although
research is still being carried out on the use of these
devices for CFS, there are trials which show their effec-
tiveness with migraine.

Fiona

Fiona, 39, is from southern England, and lives with a supportive partner. Her CFS followed a high-pressure career in publicity. Her illness came after a viral infection from which she did not fully recover. After many months with no energy, 'foggy brain', muscle pain and problems of sleep disturbance, she was forced to use a wheelchair. Eventually she was given in-patient treatment with strong MAOI (monoamine–oxidase inhibitors) drugs, which induced sleep in order to rest her central nervous system. Whilst in hospital she also received cognitive behaviour therapy (CBT).

The benefits she gained from the CBT were that she was helped to think positively about her illness. However, it was when she started to change her diet and follow the anti-candida programme that she made most progress with her symptoms. Further improvements in her 'foggy brain' came when she cut out gluten. The low gluten in oats meant that after a while she was able to reintroduce that cereal on a rotation basis.

At the same time she found a remedial yoga class. This improved her muscle function, taught her how to breathe properly, and helped her relax. Yoga gave her the feeling that she was back in control of her health and well-being. At first she needed two days' bed rest after each class, but this eventually came down to two hours, and now she is able to do yoga and feel energized and relaxed without needing rest.

Sleep problems were normalized with the use of a device to restore missing brain waves. She is convinced this device is helping because when her battery runs out without her knowledge, her sleep patterns become disturbed again, returning to normal when a new battery is inserted.

Finding a homoeopath at the end of all this treatment has been 'the icing on the cake'. She feels that homoeopathy would have been too gentle earlier on, but now it is working at a subtle level to give her more sustainable energy.

CHAPTER 8

Treating the mind and emotions

The battle to gain recognition for CFS has meant that some doctors are finally listening. But the struggle to 'prove' the physical basis of this illness has hidden from view the notion that one can speed recovery by treating the mind and the emotions too. The situation is further complicated by the fact that apart from ill-health being prompted by psychological pain or repressed emotions – something which is not a 'failure' or a cause for shame – physical illness can easily produce psychological problems. Pain, hormonal disruption, lack of sleep, despair at the loss of former capacities and anger at the loss of former relationships and lifestyles all play a part. Medical ambivalence and the reluctance to acknowledge the reality of this illness gives those with CFS every reason for anger, grief and despair.

The vital links between what we think and feel and our physical health are our hormones and neurotransmitters, made by the endocrine system in the brain. Hormones control our moods, and at a fundamental level we also affect our hormones by the way we think. Feeling low can weaken the immune system, and allows illness to take hold. This chapter looks at the many ways you can work with yourself, sometimes with the help of others, in order to heal your mind and emotions, and ultimately your body.

Underlying any techniques or therapies you select to work on your emotions, there needs to be an understanding that other therapies, as described in the last chapter, may also be necessary. It is not likely that one change or intervention will bring about an overnight cure. A more sustaining hope is one which has a realistic understanding of slow gradual improvement across many fronts.

Calming the mind

Relaxation can only be achieved with a calm mind – little or no thinking, analysing or anxiety. This can be achieved by re-examining your relationship to your mind. In Western culture we think that the thinking mind is the centre of our being. In Eastern cultures the centre, or core, is the soul, spirit or consciousness.

Dr William Collinge, in his indispensable book *Recovery from ME*, says that since in CFS your mind and its functioning can be affected by the syndrome, you can gain some power and control with the realization that you can separate yourself from your thoughts. As a result you begin to accept that the syndrome is transitory, that symptoms come and go, and that healing is possible.

The following are all necessary preconditions for calming the mind:

- a willingness to practise regularly – daily, for a specified period such as 30 minutes
- a willingness to work with your resistance – your mind will resist and prefer to remain active, and you will need to reaffirm your intention to practise regularly
- a willingness to be non-judgemental of yourself – your mind is clever at sabotaging your efforts to change it, and will try to introduce thoughts which undermine what you are trying to achieve

- the creation of the right environment – comfortable and free from distractions of people, noise and telephones

Techniques to calm the mind, focusing on the 'now', are easy to follow, but they may take time to really work. They are as follows:

- using the breath, watching the expansion and relaxation of your belly, counting the in-breath and out-breath in pairs up to ten, and starting again, or focusing on the beginning, the middle and the end of each breath
- using words or sounds – words with a calming effect, or a phrase such as 'healing now'; the method used in meditation
- using 'progressive relaxation' by focusing on various parts of your body, and relaxing them one by one

---

A simple breathing exercise

After you have regulated your breathing and relaxed your body, sitting or lying back with your eyes closed, you should focus your attention on your breath as it enters and leaves your nostrils. Focus solely on the nostrils, and the taking in and letting out of breath through them. Feel the sensations of the air going in and going out.

The sensations may change from a dull feather to itching, intense pressure, or numerous other feelings. Remember that there is no right or wrong way of doing this exercise. The focus is on the breath. If your mind starts to distract you, try counting one on inhalation and two on exhalation. If that does not work, just bring your mind back calmly and try again.

Meditation is a way of resting the mind, and the techniques used are no more than those described above. It helps, however, to be taught how to do it. The British

Holistic Medical Association publishes audio tapes for relaxation and meditation as part of its Tapes For Health series (*see* Appendix C).

One recovered PWC found that he needed to combine meditation with movement and massage. He said:

'You need to be able to reach a point where you can see yourself healthy and happy during meditation, and to be able to pour out love to yourself in a totally unconditional way.'

Visualization

This technique uses the power of your imagination to promote wellness. Some people are better at using visual images than others, who may respond more to sounds, or to stories which use suggestion. Nevertheless, it can be very relaxing to imagine yourself in a warm and beautiful place which has a special meaning to you. Some PWCs are able to imagine their immune systems mopping up free radicals, using the imagery of a battle. Others use more gentle imagery. Whatever suits you is best.

Affirmations

Affirmations are ways of talking to yourself which are positive and health promoting. They work best when you repeat them many times at different times of the day. Examples are: 'I accept myself as I am' or 'I am becoming healthy and strong.' Combined with relaxation and visualization, affirmations have helped many people change from negative ways to more positive ones.

Autogenics

Autogenics is one of the most practical stress management and relaxation techniques available. It is a medically validated series of mental exercises designed to switch off the stress 'flight and fight' response and to bring about and maintain a balance in the body–mind connection. The exercises are easy to do anywhere and at any time, but you need initial training in individual or group sessions. It involves directing your attention inwards and focusing your mind on phrases relating to different parts of the body, in the following way:

- sensations of heaviness in your body
- warmth in your arms and legs
- your calm and regular heartbeat
- your easy and natural breathing
- warmth in your abdomen
- coolness in your head

Changes of circulation and temperature occur in the areas of the body you are focusing on. Overall the technique helps with pain control, relaxation and better sleep.

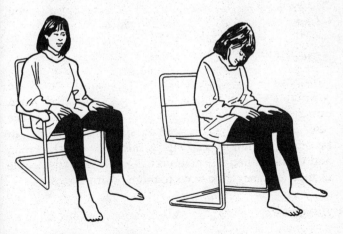

Fig. 4 Autogenic positions

Biofeedback

The use of technology in this technique to access mind and body feedback may help those who find other routes too slow. A meter is used to help you recognize your body's response, which is measured by electrodes held in your hand or taped to your head. The meters pick up the difference between feeling tense and feeling relaxed, so that you gradually learn to sense the difference for yourself, and are able to effect positive change.

Counselling and psychotherapy

Counselling is about talking about yourself and your problems to a trained and experienced listener. Through this you are helped to express your feelings, and to understand your situation, and enabled to work out solutions. This is especially helpful to PWCs who may be reluctant to burden carers who are already providing a lot of physical support and coping with feelings of their own.

However, you should make sure that any therapist you consult in any of the counselling therapies has some understanding of CFS beforehand. Otherwise they may work solely on the psychological level. Counsellors are available in many primary care health centres.

Psychotherapy concentrates more on tackling the deeper, often hidden, underlying causes of what troubles you, although the differences between the two are not always clear, especially in the USA. Again, you should check that the psychotherapist understands the multicausal nature of CFS, and the relapsing and remitting nature of the illness.

Most of the psychological therapies you are likely to encounter fall into three broad categories:

- psychodynamic therapies, which seek understanding by extensively exploring unconscious feelings
- humanistic therapies, which seek to help clients find their own answers
- cognitive/behavioural therapies, which help clients to identify and reach goals without looking at the causes of the behaviour, helping to change the way the client views the world

Many therapists and counsellors take elements from each of these approaches, although some stay fairly rigidly within their original discipline.

Some PWCs gain help from co-counselling, a reciprocal method of self-help, although they may need other therapies at different stages. After the initial training cost it is free, because it involves you giving someone else as much counselling as you are receiving. One of its advantages is that it avoids the dependency problems that can arise with one-way counselling. However, it is only suitable for those who have the energy to return what they have received. Another pitfall of co-counselling is that in amateur hands it may fail to help the participants make progress, encouraging them to focus on the symptoms rather than taking a broader perspective.

Hypnotherapy

Hypnotherapy, or hypnosis, is a technique well supported by research, in which trained specialists gain access to unconscious or repressed mental and emotional problems. Through deep relaxation, the conscious mind is turned off. The hypnotherapist, when properly trained, can work with you to help you 'get in touch' with whatever causes your problem. Some of the most successful hypnotherapists are also trained in counselling or psychotherapy. The reason they also use hypnotherapy is because it can speed up finding the source of the problem, and is a very effective route to deep relaxation. It is possible to learn self-hypnosis as a way of relaxation and tension release. However, the use of hypnosis as a form of entertainment has deflected attention from its health value in responsible and skilled hands, and it is important to choose a therapist carefully (*see* chapter 11).

T'ai chi ch'uan

T'ai chi ch'uan has often been called 'meditation in motion'. It is thought to have been developed out of a blend of Taoist philosophy and the martial arts in 11th-century China. It involves a series of slow movements which encourage energy flow. You could prepare yourself for this therapy by reading *The Way of Energy* by Master Lam Kam Chuen (*see* Appendix B). With this book you can learn exercises which can be done even if you are bedridden.

Yoga

Yoga is suitable for all ages and levels of fitness, and is one of the most complete mind–body therapies there is. It is particularly recommended for PWCs. You will be taught the correct way to breathe and given gentle stretching movements and postures which will gradually extend your suppleness and energy levels. Yoga will also help your mental state, with profound psychological benefits.

The Yoga for Health Foundation (*see* Appendix A) in the UK runs special courses for CFS, for all levels of experience. Finding a local class should not be difficult, although it is best to find a teacher who understands the particular need to go very slowly.

Alexander technique

F Mathias Alexander was an actor at the turn of the century who had problems with his voice whilst on stage. He discovered that the cause was tension in his neck and throat. The technique he developed helps to stop old habits, using the mind–body connection to let go of tension and excess muscle effort. A large part of CFS seems to be the feeling that the body is totally at odds with itself. Alexander helps you to lessen the load, reduce fatigue and improve general well-being. It can also help the practice of yoga. Although it is sometimes taught in groups, it is preferable with CFS if it is taught individually.

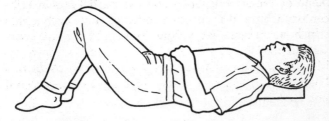

Fig. 5 A relaxation posture in the Alexander technique

Graham

Graham, an active, 'outdoors' person with a successful career, became bedridden after a long period of decreasing energy and reduced ability to concentrate. For three years he could not read, walk upstairs or even talk for very long. When he started to lose his sight, he agreed to be admitted to an acute psychiatric ward under a psychiatrist who specialized in CFS. He became worse, and after five weeks he experienced what he describes as a 'breakdown' of emotional and physical release, after which his recovery started.

During the next three years he had psychotherapy, and took up t'ai chi ch'uan and yoga, as well as a whole range of expressive therapies and activities. He started to experience severe pain in the neck and shoulders and over the next two years went through two major relapses involving total incapacity. They lasted many months. Then he was introduced to the Chinese internal energy exercise system called *zhan zhuang*, or 'standing like a tree'. This is the most powerful form of chi kung. After a few minutes' practise he felt some increase in energy, but pain limited the amount he could do. With time, he was able to increase his tolerance and made good progress, until he was spending several hours each day on the exercises.

He also took up meditation, using the simple technique of maintaining an awareness of breathing, again building up to several hours each day. During the course of a meditation retreat, he experienced what he describes as 'instances of indescribable peace and understanding. I became aware of the reasons for my illness and could explain my subsequent recovery in terms of my own "mind state", gradually moving from negative to positive and finally coming under my own control.'

A second meditation retreat initiated a physical release of tensions in his body. He started to feel energy flows in his limbs, and suppleness and strength returned. He developed a system of self-massage whereby he pressed all areas of his body, searching out for painful and tender areas, which with further pressure gradually dispersed.

He is now able to resume jogging, swimming, cycling and even mountaineering. With recovery he knew that he faced the risk of change in all areas of his life. He has not returned to his former work. Instead he hopes to help others find their own route to change.

This chapter has looked at techniques which you can learn to help your mind and body towards recovery. The key to self-healing seems to be a quiet, conducive environment, conscious muscular relaxation, awareness of breathing, quietening of the mind, positive mental imagery and free emotional expression. It is up to you to find the time and the commitment to put it into practice.

Avoiding the pitfalls of working with the mind–body connection

- Do not blame yourself. Take responsibility for the here and now.
- Hope is not unrealistic, but it should sit beside a realistic understanding of what is involved.
- Emotions should not be seen as negative or positive. Rather they are an expression of your life force, and should be recognized, whatever they are. Repressing negative emotion means that you delay acceptance of who you are.
- Avoid performance anxiety and fear of failure when trying new techniques and therapies.
- Do not place all your hope for recovery on one thing. It is difficult not knowing what to blame when an illness has more than one cause. Do not blame yourself. Do the best you can and be patient.

CHAPTER 9

Treating the life force

Some therapies work at an energetic and vibrational level. Vibrational medicine sees the body as a series of interacting fields of energy. This perspective looks at the body as an electrical circuit. It also acknowledges the role of other energies which are difficult to measure, such as psychic energy.

Acupuncture

Acupuncture originated in China more than 4,000 years ago, and now there are thought to be around 3 million practitioners worldwide. In the West more and more doctors are training in this therapy because they are impressed with its ability to control pain and cure addictions. Some operations can be performed with acupuncture without the use of anaesthetics.

The treatment uses very fine steel needles, usually painless on insertion, to stimulate the body's subtle energy (known as *chi* in Chinese) at any of some 361 specific points along 14 meridians or energetic pathways within the body. Some practitioners combine acupuncture with the use of Chinese herbs. Acupressure uses finger pressure (and sometimes elbow, knee or heel pressure) instead of needles.

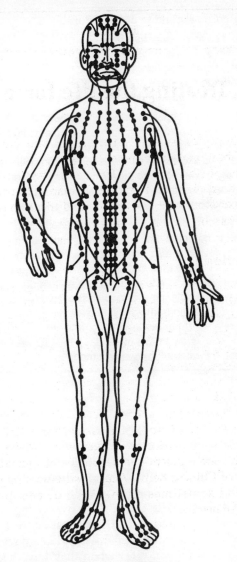

Fig. 6 The acupuncture energy meridians

How PWCs respond to acupuncture

Responses to acupuncture vary enormously. In 1996 a small survey by the British charity Action for ME found that whereas some members had gained enormously, others had suffered a relapse or felt no difference. Here are some quotes from those with positive experiences.

I have found acupuncture to be very helpful in alleviating the more distressing symptoms, particularly difficulty in standing up due to exhaustion and pain, aching in joints, general flu-like malaise, over-sensitivity to noise, memory loss and impaired concentration, intense cold during the night and insomnia. Although the treatment has not made the condition go away it has made an enormous difference to the quality of my life on a day-to-day basis.

There is no doubt that acupuncture improved my physical energy levels. It also helped reduce my anxiety. When the needles went in I felt like a radiator that has just had its valves opened to release pressure. Within 30 seconds my fists would unclench and I would feel so relaxed. As soon as I stopped the treatment and went on holiday I had a bad relapse. After resuming acupuncture I stabilized within two weeks. Now I have maintained my progress despite stopping treatment for over six months.

Healing

Healing is often wrongly referred to as 'faith healing', but it is not necessary to believe in its benefits for it to work. It is a simple and safe way of affecting the body by the use of touch, or by passing the hands over the body. Experiments have also shown that healing can work from a distance, with thoughts or by looking at a photograph. This is the most difficult aspect of healing to understand, but experiments with plants have shown a difference in growth rates when they have been on the receiving end of distance healing.

Those who are sensitive to healing feel changes of temperature, either intense heat or, more rarely, sudden cold. Others feel a tingling, like electricity, or sudden shifts of energy through their bodies. But you do not have to feel anything for it to work. Healers work in different ways, but most are able to feel changes in the body at a vibrational level, and work to unblock stagnant energy by transferring energy from their bodies to the client's.

Some PWCs are helped by regular visits to healers, relaxing and gaining renewed energy. If you do not gain anything from healing that is not your failure. It just means that you should try another healer or work with a different therapy which suits you better.

Therapeutic touch

Therapeutic touch or TT is a modern version of healing, and is used particularly in the USA, where to call oneself a healer using psychic or supernatural powers is illegal in many states. Nevertheless, TT shares the same belief in the transfer of energy through touch, and its use is increasing by nurses in clinics and hospitals in the USA.

Reiki

Reiki (pronounced 'ray-key') is a technique involving the laying on of hands, and is believed to have originated in Tibet thousands of years ago. It was rediscovered in the mid-1800s by a Japanese monk, and came to the West in the late 1930s. It works on the basis of channelled energy, an unseen universal energy which the reiki practitioner draws through the body and out through the hands to the recipient, usually felt as heat. At first adverse reactions are common, and they are welcomed. Reiki is useful for PWCs because, with training, it can be self-administered.

Anthea

After developing myocarditis (a viral infection) Anthea went on to develop CFS, with all the symptoms of energy loss, brain fogginess, muscle pain and continual headaches. She had a six-week period in hospital, unable to get up for more than two hours a day. A year later she tried various antidepressants, none of which helped. Starting in therapy did help, however. Looking back she feels this was the turning point. 'Sorting out old emotional baggage wasn't easy, but I came to understand, and in time change, my behaviour patterns and to learn the lessons that enabled me to start moving towards recovery.'

Forced to go back to work because she lived on her own with no other means of support, she worked three days a week in order to take four days to recover. At the same time she experimented with any treatment she could find, including acupuncture, homoeopathy, nutrition and a device to correct brain frequencies. The latter helped her to work. The treatment which made the most difference to her health, however, was reiki.

The first three sessions brought on cleansing and detoxifying reactions which, without the encouragement of her therapist, would have caused her to give up. However, after the fourth treatment she noticed that she could push herself and not suffer any consequences in energy drain or relapse, as before. 'Now I was only ordinarily and healthily tired and this was terrific. Gradually I came to accept that the unbelievable could be permanent.' Anthea knows that she is not back to 100 per cent of her former self, but she has probably reached 90 per cent. She has now moved on to learn the technique for herself, using it in addition for minor aches and pains, and on friends. She calls this gift of self-healing her path back to the real world.

Homoeopathy

Homoeopathy takes dilute and minute substances which cause illness, and through a process of shaking them vigorously several times, increases their potency. These substances can then be used to cure illness. This may sound strange, but despite much medical scepticism, it works, and is safe. In the UK it is the oldest natural therapy available free on the National Health Service, through doctors who are also trained as homoeopaths.

Although some homoeopaths have tried to show that it is effective for CFS, there is not much evidence, anecdotal or otherwise, to show that it works on its own. However, it can be useful when the PWC is starting to recover (*see* the case study on pp81–2).

Reflexology

In this technique, the feet are seen as a map of the body, connected to it via ten vertical lines of energy rather like the Chinese meridians or energy channels. Crystalline deposits beneath the skin indicate an imbalance, and massaging the relevant zone on the foot (*see* p100) can bring relief to the organ or area affected. It is particularly helpful when someone is in too much pain to be treated on the spot itself, or when the deep organs need help.

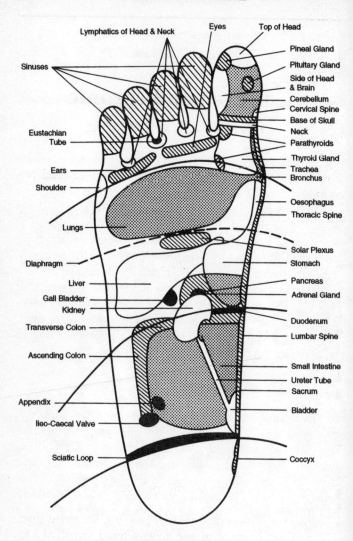

Fig. 7 Reflexology zones on the right foot

CHAPTER 10

Children and chronic fatigue syndrome

The most common symptoms in children with CFS are as follows:

- abnormal tiredness, exhaustion, fatigue, often with no loss of motivation, and waking from a night sleep feeling exhausted
- acute onset with temperature and/or sore throat and lymph node enlargement
- muscle pain and/or tenderness
- impaired concentration
- headache (persistent, and not responsive to painkillers)
- altered sleep pattern, ie changes from normality
- aching/feeling 'ill all over'
- circulatory disturbances, feeling hot but cold to the touch, freezing hands on a warm day, or a hot and cold feeling to the body simultaneously
- disturbance of memory, concentrating ability, ability to name common objects
- anorexia/nausea
- severe chest or stomach ache for most of the day
- limb and/or backache
- blurring of vision or difficulty reading for more than 10 minutes because of eye ache, altered sensitivity to light, altered sensitivity to sound
- persistent change of bowel habit compared to normal state

- standing still being considerably more tiring than walking

The most severe forms of the disease are thought to be more common in children than in adults. It is the neurological symptoms which are often worse, such as:

- dizziness
- mental confusion
- unremitting headache
- severe shaking episodes
- sensitivity to light
- difficulty in swallowing
- hypersensitivity to noise

Research to show recovery rates is scarce. There is anecdotal evidence, however, which suggests that children do recover, though they may need to be careful not to overdo things for a long time afterwards. Essential for progress is a supportive situation of acceptance by the medical team. Parents also need support. The level of care needed for the child is very high; some children are unable to feed themselves and have difficulty swallowing, and others are unable to get out of bed unaided.

Prevalence and duration

In the USA one study suggested that there are around 2 children per 1,000 with CFS, although the criteria used have since been found to be too narrowly defined. In the UK it has been estimated that there are as many as 25,000. A recent study by consultant microbiologist Dr Betty Dowsett and Jane Colby of 1,098 UK schools over a five-year period found that 51 per cent of the long-term sickness was attributable to CFS. The average prevalence was 70 per 100,000 children.

CFS is not often found in children under five, and

between five and 12 the start of the illness is more likely to be gradual. Puberty is the usual time of onset, and from this time on CFS is more likely to start following a viral infection.

American data suggests that, unlike adults, in children the sexes are equally represented, but once over puberty girls are more likely to develop CFS than boys – one survey of a consultant's patients found that whereas 16 were male, 38 were female. The duration of the illness for these children varied from four months to seven years.

Some children become worse as a result of being pushed back to school too soon, because there may be a strictly limited amount of energy for the whole day and rest may be needed after travel or movement around the school building, or after mental or physical effort. Naturally, absences cause more pressure because of the need to catch up on work on return to school, which can precipitate a relapse.

Diagnosis

CFS in children is even more controversial than in adults, in that their reporting of symptoms is often assumed to have a psychological origin, with the result that they are encouraged to exercise or return to school. It is assumed that there is some secondary gain from illness in the opportunity it provides to skip school. But the key features of school phobia are that the child is active in the home but not at school, with no physical illness, and that separation anxiety or fear of bullying at school are the main underlying factors.

Somatic complaints are common among children, and because of this, and the inconsistent nature of the symptoms, it is understandable that paediatricians sometimes misdiagnose CFS in children. Dr Frank

Albrecht and Rebecca Moore point out in a CFIDS Youth Alliance paper (*Why Children with CFS Are Often Overlooked*, April 1996) that part of the problem is that the children themselves often decide that their symptoms are too normal to mention, or so strange that they should be hidden. Children are less sure of their abilities than adults, and their symptoms may manifest as progressive school difficulties. In addition, children do not have the kind of autonomy or assertiveness needed to stand up to adults who do not believe them, and tend to believe that what adults tell them must be true. So if they are told they are not ill they try to believe it.

Educational and social pressures

One factor which is often overlooked is that severely affected CFS children are unable to cope with full-time schooling due to the combination of physical fatigue and cognitive dysfunction, something which is not the case in most other chronic childhood illnesses. Home tutoring on a one-to-one basis, which is gradually increased as the child improves, is sometimes a better option, with an eventual return to school on a part-time basis, building up to full time with careful management and supervision.

Many doctors, however, are concerned about the damage to the child arising from the social isolation of missing school when home tutoring is given. This is a very real problem: because the disease is often severe in children, it usually results in a loss of contact with friends, which can lead to problems of self-esteem and difficulties with relationships. When they become ill adults can often look back to achievements in work, or past pleasure or satisfaction in other areas of their lives. Children live in the moment, and have few such memories to fall back on. Their future seems to be cut short because of illness. Often vital years of education are missed, along with essential practice in social skills, and independence. The question of whether medical concern to get the child back into school as soon as possible is appropriate is an ongoing debate, and is underpinned by different views of causation and management. Certainly, doctors' fears about complete inactivity should be taken seriously. Some form of movement is necessary each day, rather than complete inactivity and total bed rest.

However, where school phobia is incorrectly used as a diagnosis it is often difficult for the doctor to work cooperatively with the family. The family's feeling that something else is wrong other than avoidance of school is seen by the medical authorities as obstructing appropriate treatment – teaching the child to overcome whatever family dynamics are keeping him or her at home, and encouraging activity. The parents come to be seen as the main stumbling block to effective psychiatric care and eventual rehabilitation. There is a case to be made for providing some families with therapy and support, where CFS may not be the correct diagnosis or where coping with CFS has heightened stress and fear to a level which sends the child into a downward spiral of ill-health.

In CFS the child becomes dependent, powerless and seemingly at the mercy of an illness which even adults do not understand. Children can be profoundly affected by the attitudes of those around them. Picking up on fear and pessimism can result in a deep sense of hopelessness. Turning that around, giving back a sense of control and working in partnership with all the agencies involved can be enormously beneficial. This is essential because otherwise the grief at the inability to learn and the loss of friends can overwhelm the child. This can lead to irritability or withdrawal and occasionally to suicidal thoughts and depression.

It is important for parents to help their child to feel in control. Children need to know that they are being heard, and that nothing is being done to them which they fear may cause them pain and relapse. Whatever support and treatment is used, it should be part of a programme which the child or young adult has agreed to and helped to put together. One of the problems for children comes with management. They have greater difficulty in accepting limitations, and in understanding the time it may take to recover from CFS.

Dr Alan Franklin, a British paediatrician with a substantial case-load of children with CFS, has seen many children who have lost confidence in medical advisors and others when these problems are not recognized. Another consequence is an overdependence on their parents, which medical personnel could be prone to interpret as the cause of the CFS rather than the result. Parents are assumed to encourage this dependence to satisfy their own needs. But in fact, most of them express a need to be protective initially in order to defend their child against what they fear to be inappropriate treatment, based on their experience of caring for the child 24 hours a day. This is not helped by the fact that CFS comes and goes, and there is bound to be a lot of fear about relapse and overdoing things.

Jessica

Jessica had a severe stomach bug when she was 11 years old, causing her to be ill for over five weeks. Shortly after recovering, tonsillitis and glandular fever symptoms developed. The year after she returned to school, she became ill again, this time much more seriously and had to stay in bed until the afternoon. The energy she used in getting up, dressing and going downstairs did not leave her enough to do anything else for the rest of the day. The pain was extreme, and her head was so heavy that she wanted to put it on her arms; it was aching all the time. A paediatrician diagnosed school phobia and maternal anxiety. 'All I remember is being absolutely scared stiff because I knew then that I would not get any support at all. And I knew that what he was saying was totally wrong.' She improved with another doctor who was more sympathetic, but went on to push herself at school too soon and had another relapse. The school tried to insist that she return full time or not at all. The stress this brought on caused severe migraines and she spiralled down into complete relapse. A visit to a psychiatrist produced more psychological questioning and a prescription to do more exercises. When she refused to carry on with this because of the increased pain and disability that resulted, she was made to discharge herself, with no further contact with her doctors, except a supportive GP.

The turning point came with the involvement of an educational psychologist. 'She listened and she accepted what I was saying was the truth, which was what I needed.' A team of professionals was brought together – a physiotherapist, a hydrotherapist, the GP, the school doctor and her tutors – and Jessica was allowed to chair the meetings. For the first time she was put in control of what was to happen to her. She feels that this prevented her from sinking into depression. Before, she had felt that the illness was controlling her.

Jessica's story is told in her own words in *ME: The New Plague* by Jane Colby.

The British charity, Action for ME, has published a Children's Charter, which is a set of guidelines for the many professionals involved in the management of childhood CFS. This could be a useful tool if you need to ensure good communication between the various agencies and professionals caring for your child. You may also need advice on how to secure home tutoring when school is not possible.

CHAPTER 11

How to choose and find a natural therapist

One of the most important things to bear in mind is that it is not just a question of finding the right therapy and the right therapist. It is also a question of timing, and how you combine different therapies or interventions. Some therapies may not be effective in the early stages when your mental attitude may be negative. On the other hand, your mental attitude could change as a result of your relationship with a particular therapist, allowing you to open up to the possibility of change. You may also need to concentrate on the self-help aspects, pacing and living within your energy limits, before searching for outside solutions.

The therapeutic encounter and permission to hope

Because in Western society we invest doctors and therapists with the power to heal, we are culturally tuned to internalize their view of our situation, and whether they believe they can help. This affects the quality of the relationship and how we perceive our chances of recovery. Moreover, the emotional component of illness is often, understandably, denied or avoided by doctors and practitioners. This is because of difficult feelings such as fear, anger, isolation, despair and grief. Patients who are allowed to express these feelings and are listened to have a better chance of recovery.

Without that openness to the reality of chronic illness in emotional terms, PWCs are vulnerable to pessimism (which is realistic if feelings are cut off) from the people in whom they invest the power to heal. Sometimes, rather than searching for others' permission, we need to to give it to ourselves. Discovering what we need from within ourselves may in the end be the most valuable lesson to learn.

Finding a therapist

It is much easier now to find the right therapist than it was even a few years ago – but it is still not easy enough. The sheer variety of therapies is bewildering in itself and in many countries natural therapists are still not fully organized. There is no shortage of directories and advertisements but it's difficult to assess the reliability of their information. So how do you find a therapist you can trust?

Starting the search: local sources

As we have seen, many of the natural therapies high-lighted in this book have their roots in antiquity. Some have existed for as long as human beings have lived on Earth, and finding a good practitioner has been a matter of tuning in to the community 'bush telegraph'. Word of mouth is still the best way to find the right practitioner.

Speak to anyone whose opinion you respect, especially a fellow sufferer. (You will also want to know who should be avoided, and which therapies might not help you at all.) If this does not work there are several other ways you can try.

Doctors' clinics and medical centres

If you need help urgently you must see your family

doctor. If you ask about natural therapies at your first appointment, be prepared to hear anything from a dire warning to a recommendation that you try a natural therapist in view of the fact that there is nothing to lose.

Natural health centres

Your nearest natural health centre should be happy to advise you. Your first impressions will often be a good guide to the quality of service they provide. Are the staff well informed and friendly? Is the place clean and comfortable? Does the atmosphere make you feel comfortable from the moment you walk in? It should. It matters. You are bringing them your trust and your custom and both should be treated with the utmost respect.

A good centre should have plenty of information explaining the therapies and introducing the practitioners. In a well-run practice the receptionist or owner will know all about the different therapies on offer. It's a bad sign if they don't.

You may still be unsure after your first impressions whether to book in or not. If so, ask to meet the person who might be treating you, just to test the waters. This should be possible, even in a busy practice.

Don't start off by telling your full life history, but some practices do offer you this opportunity during a free consultation – usually 15 minutes – just to see whether you have come to the right place or not.

Local practitioners

Practitioners tend to know who's who in the area, even in therapies other than their own. So if you know, say, a reflexologist but want a homoeopath, ask for a recommendation. The same applies if you know a practitioner socially and so don't want to consult him or her professionally. Practitioners are usually happy to recommend someone else in the same field.

Healthfood stores and alternative bookshops

The staff in these kinds of shops often have a good local knowledge as well as an interest in the subject of natural therapies. The shop may well have a noticeboard with local practitioners' business cards on it. Remember, though, the most experienced and well-established practitioners don't need this kind of advertising, so you might miss them altogether if you don't actually check up by asking.

Other sources of local knowledge

Don't forget that your local pharmacist often has contacts with both conventional and natural therapists. The local library or information centre may be another good source of contact, especially for finding self-help or support groups.

Computers (using a modem) can provide information via the Internet system and other sources worth trying are health farms, beauty therapists and citizens' advice bureaux.

Wider sources of information

If you have no luck on a local level, don't give up – there are several more leads you can follow up at a national level.

'Umbrella' organizations

The natural therapies are increasingly coming together under 'umbrella' organizations that represent a therapy or range of therapies nationally under one banner or heading. These national umbrella organizations have lists of registered and approved practitioners, and in the case of the more established therapies (such as chiropractic) have their own regulatory bodies already in place.

It is better to phone than to write or fax because this should give you a good idea of how well organized the group is. You may find that the group you are contacting has several different associations under its banner. A small charge may be made for each association's register but if you can afford it get the lot and then make up your own mind.

Newspapers, magazines and local directories

Many therapists advertise. If you find local practitioners this way it's a good idea to talk to them and check them out first.

Checking professional organizations

Some organizations are genuine groups that really keep a check on their members, while others seem to spring up like weeds, apparently interested only in collecting membership fees and giving themselves credibility. This section helps you do your own weeding.

Why do professional organizations exist?

The purposes of governing bodies for natural therapies are:

- to keep up-to-date lists of their members so you can check whether someone is really on their list
- to protect you by making sure that their members are fully trained, licensed and insured against accident, negligence and malpractice
- to give you someone to complain to if you are unhappy with any aspect of treatment you have received, and you can't sort the matter out with your therapist
- to protect their members by giving good ethical and legal advice

- to represent their members when laws which might affect them are being made
- to work towards improvements in education for their members both before and after qualifying
- to work towards greater awareness of the benefit of each therapy in conventional medical circles
- to improve public awareness of the benefit of each therapy

Questions to ask professional organizations
A good organization will publish clear and simple information on its status and purposes along with its membership list. As they don't all do this you may find it useful to contact them again on receiving your list to ask the following:

- When was the association founded? (You may be reassured to hear it has been around for 50 years. If the association is new, however, don't reject it out of hand. Ask why it was formed – it may be innovative.)
- How many members does it have? (Size reflects public demand, as few therapists could survive in a therapy if there was no call for it. The bigger organizations generally have a better track record and greater public acceptance, but a small association may just reflect the fact that the therapy is very specialized or still in its infancy – not necessarily a bad thing.)
- When was the therapy that it represents started?
- Is it a charity or educational trust – with a proper constitution, management committee and published accounts – or is it a private limited company? (Charities have to be non-profitmaking, work in the public interest and be open to inspection at any time. Private companies don't.)
- Is it part of a larger network of organizations? (If so, this implies it is interested in progress by consensus

with other groups, and not just in furthering its own aims. By and large, groups that go their own way are more suspect than those that join in.)

- Does the organization have a code of ethics (upholding standards of professional behaviour) and disciplinary procedures? If so, what are they?
- How do its members gain admission to its register? Is it linked to only one school? (Beware of associations whose heads are also head of the school they represent: unbiased help may be in short supply with this type of 'one-man band'.)
- Do members have to have proof of professional indemnity insurance? This should cover:
  - accidental damage to yourself or your property while you are on the practitioner's work premises
  - negligence (either the failure of the practitioner to exercise the 'duty of care' owed to you, or his or her falling below the standards of clinical competence demanded by his or her qualifications, bringing about an overall worsening of your problem)
  - malpractice (a 'falling from grace' over professional conduct, involving, for example, dishonesty, sexual misconduct or breach of confidence – your personal details should *never* be discussed with a third person without your permission)

Checking training and qualifications

If you have reassured yourself so far but are still puzzled by what the training actually involves, ask a few more questions:

- How long is the training?
- Is it full or part time?
- If it is part time but shorter than a full-time course leading to the same qualifications, does the time spent

at lectures and in clinic add up to the same as a full-time course overall? (In other words, is it a short cut?)
- Does it include seeing patients under supervision at a college clinic and in real practices?
- What do the initials after the therapist's name mean? Do they denote simply membership of an organization or do they indicate in-depth study?
- Are the qualifications recognized? If so, by whom? (This is becoming more relevant as the therapy organizations group together and start to form state-recognized registers in many countries. But the really important thing to know is if the qualifications are recognized by an independent outside assessment authority.)

Making the choice

Making the final choice is a matter of using a combination of common sense and intuition, and finding the resolution to give someone a try. Don't forget that the most important part of the whole process is your resolve to feel better, to have more control over your state of health, and hopefully to see an improvement in your condition. The next most important part is that you feel comfortable with your chosen therapist.

What is it like seeing a natural therapist?

Since most natural therapists, even in those countries with state health systems, still work privately, there is no established common pattern.

Although they may all share more or less a belief in the principles outlined in chapter 6, you are liable to come across individuals from all walks of life. You will find as much variety in dress, thinking and behaviour as there are fashions, ranging from the formal and sophisticated to the absolutely informal.

Equally, you will find their premises very different. Some will present a 'brass plaque' image, working in a clinic with a receptionist and brisk efficiency, while others will see you in their living room surrounded by plants and domestic clutter.

Remember, though, that while image may be some indication of status, it is little guarantee of ability. You are as likely to find a therapist of quality working from home as in a formal clinic.

Some characteristics, though, and probably the most important ones, are common to all natural therapists:

- They will give you far more time than you are used to with a family doctor. An initial consultation will rarely last less than an hour, and is often longer. They will ask you all about yourself so they can form a proper understanding of what makes you tick and what may be the fundamental cause(s) of your problem.
- You will have to pay for any remedies they prescribe, and they may well sell you these from their own stocks. They will also charge you for their time – though many therapists offer reduced fees for deserving cases or for people who genuinely cannot afford the full fee.

Sensible precautions

- Be sceptical of anyone who 'guarantees' you a cure. No one (not even doctors) can do that.
- Query any attempt to book you in for a course of treatment. Your response to any natural therapy is highly individual. Of course, if the practice is a busy one, booking ahead for one or two sessions might be

sensible. You should be able to cancel without penalty any sessions which prove unnecessary (but remember to give at least 24 hours' notice: some practitioners will charge you if you don't give enough notice).

- No ethical therapist will ask for fees in advance of treatment unless for special tests or medicines – and even this is unusual. If you are asked for 'down payments' of any sort, ask exactly what they are for. If you don't like the reasons, don't pay.

- Be wary if you are not asked about your existing medication and try to give precise answers when you are asked. Be especially wary if the therapist tells you to stop or change any medically prescribed drug without talking to your doctor first. (A responsible doctor should also be happy to discuss you and your medication with a therapist.)

- Note the quality of the therapist's touch if you choose any of the relaxation or manipulation techniques, such as massage, aromatherapy or osteopathy. It should never be lingering or suggestive. If, for any reason, the therapist wants to touch you on the breasts or genitals, your permission should be sought first.

- If the practitioner is of the opposite sex you are entitled to have someone of your choice in the room at the same time. Be immediately suspicious if this is not allowed. Ethical therapists will not refuse this sort of request, and if they do, it is probably best to have nothing more to do with them.

What to do if things go wrong

A practitioner is in a position of trust, and is charged with a duty of care to you at all times. It does not mean you are 'entitled' to a 'cure' just because you've paid for treatment, but if you feel you are being treated unfairly, incompetently or unethically, you have several options:

- Tackle the matter at the source of the problem, with your practitioner, either verbally or in writing.
- If he or she works in a place such as a clinic, health farm or sports centre, tell the management. They also have a duty to protect the public and should treat complaints seriously and discreetly.
- Contact the practitioner's professional organization. It should have an independent panel that investigates complaints fully and disciplines its members.
- If the offence committed is a criminal one report it to the police (but be prepared for the problem of proving one person's word against another's).
- If you feel compensation is due see a lawyer for advice.

Short of a public court case, the worst thing for a truly incompetent or unethical practitioner is bad publicity. Tell everyone about your experiences. People only need to hear the same sort of comments from a few different sources and the practitioner will probably sink without trace. Before you do so, though, try the other measures first and give yourself time to consider things calmly. Vengeance is not very healing.

A word of warning Don't make malicious allegations without good reason. Such actions are themselves a criminal offence in most countries and you could end up in more trouble than the practitioner.

Summary

The reality is that there are few crooks or charlatans in natural therapy. Despite the myth, there is little real money in it unless the therapist is very busy – and the chances are high that a busy therapist is a good one. Remember that no one can know everything and no specialist qualified in any field has to get 100 per cent in the exams to be able to practice. Perfection is an ideal, not a reality, and to err is human.

It is very much for this reason that taking control of your own health is perhaps the single most important lesson underlying this book. Taking control means taking responsibility for the choices you make, and this is one of the most significant factors in successful treatment.

APPENDIX A

Useful addresses

The following list of organizations is for information only and does not imply any endorsement, nor do the organizations listed necessarily agree with the views expressed in this book.

CFS (ME) Associations

INTERNATIONAL

CFS Electronic Newsletter
CFS-NEWS home page:
http://www.alternatives.com/cfs-news/index.htm
NIHLIST Listserv on Internet or
Roger Burns at Internet
CFS-NEWS@LIST.NIK.GOV
Tel: 1-202-966-8738

WECAN
Worldwide Electronic
CFIDS/ME Action Network
Mary M Schweitzer
Steering Committee, WECAN
WECAN
PO Box 805
Hockessin
DE 19707-0805
Tel: 610-519-7403
For more information and membership details
Web: http://www.community-care-org.uk/ME/wecan.html

American network
AACFS home page:
http://weber.u.washington.edu/~dedra/aacfs;.html

European Network
ME-NET:
http://www.dds.nl/~me-net
ME-WEB:
http://www.dds.nl/~me-net/meweb
Action for ME and Chronic
Fatigue:
http://www.afme.org.uk

For those without access to E-mail and Websites:

ME BBS Mailing Service
4 Twain Avenue
Stenhousemuir
Larbert
Stirlingshire FK5 4HL
Tel/Fax: 01324 554203
This service prints out and mails monthly information and research results on CFS(ME) from Web pages across the world.

AUSTRALIA

ANZYMES Victoria
PO Box 7
Moonee Ponds
Victoria, 3039
Australia

NEW ZEALAND

ANZYMES (NZ) INC
PO Box 35-429
Browns Bay
Auckland 10
New Zealand

NORTH AMERICA

The CFIDS Association of America, Inc.
PO Box 220398
Charlotte
NC 28222-0398
Tel: 1-800-442-3437
Fax: 704/365-9755

National CFS Association
3521 Broadway-Suite 222
Kansas City, 64111
Missouri
USA

SOUTH AFRICA

ME Association of South Africa
PO Box 461
Hillcrest 3650
Natal
South Africa

UK AND EIRE

Action for ME and Chronic Fatigue
PO Box 1302
Wells
Somerset BA5 1YE
Tel: 01749 670799
Fax: 01749 672561

The ME Association
Stanhope House
High Street
Stanford-le-Hope
Essex SS17 0HA
Tel: 01375 642466
Fax: 01375 360256

National ME Centre
Harold Wood Hospital
Gubbins Lane
Harold Wood
Romford
Essex RM3 0BE
Tel: 01708 378050
Patient referral treatment centre

Westcare
155 Whiteladies Road
Clifton
Bristol BS8 2RF
Tel: 0117 923 9341
Fax: 0117 923 9347
Rehabilitation courses for CFS (ME)

Natural medicine organizations

AUSTRALIA

Australian Natural Therapists Association
PO Box 308
Melrose Park
South Australia 5039
Tel: 618297 9533
Fax: 618297 0003

Australian Traditional Medicine Society
PO Box 442

or

Suite 3
First Floor
120 Blaxland Road
Ryde
New South Wales 2112
Australia
Tel: 612 808 2825
Fax: 612 809 7570

NORTH AMERICA

American Academy of Medical Preventics
6151 West Century Boulevard
Suite 1114
Los Angeles
California 90045, USA
Tel: 213 645 5350

American Association of Naturopathic Physicians
2800 East Madison Street
Suite 200
Seattle
Washington 98102, USA

or

PO Box 20386
Seattle
Washington 98102, USA
Tel: 206 323 7610
Fax: 206 323 7612

American Holistic Medical Association
4101 Lake Boone Trail, Suite 201
Raleigh
North Carolina 27607, USA
Tel: 919 787 5146
Fax: 919 787 4916

Canadian Holistic Medical Association
700 Bay Street
PO Box 13205, Suite 604
Toronto
Ontario M5G 1Z6, Canada
Tel: 416 5999 0447

UK AND EIRE

British Association for Counselling
1 Regent Place
Rugby
Warwickshire CV21 2PJ
Tel: 01788 578328/9

British Complementary Medicine Association
39 Prestbury Road
Pitville
Cheltenham
Gloucestershire GL52 2PT
Tel: 01242 226770
Fax: 01242 226778
Umbrella organization representing organizations outside CCAM

British Holistic Medical Association
Rowland Thomas House
Royal Shrewsbury Hospital
South
Shrewsbury
Shropshire SY3 8XF
Tel: 01743 261155
Association of medical professionals working for changes in attitudes and approaches in the National Health Service.

British Homoeopathic Association
27 Devonshire Street
London W1N 1RJ
Tel: 0171 935 2163
Members are medically trained practitioners. Send SAE for information and list of members.

Colonics International Association
50A Morrish Road
London SW2 4EG

Council for Complementary and Alternative Medicine (CCAM)
Park House, Suite D
206–208 Latimer Road
London W10 6RE
Tel: 0181 968 3862
Fax: 0181 968 3469

Institute for Complementary Medicine
PO Box 194
London SE16 1QZ
Tel: 0171 237 5165
Fax: 0171 237 5175

International Academy of Oral Medicine and Toxicology
72 Harley Street
London W1N 1AE
Tel: 0171 580 3168

National Institute of Medical Herbalists
9 Palace Gate
Exeter
Devon EX1 1JA

Natural Medicines Society
Edith Lewis House
Ilkeston
Derbyshire DE7 8EJ

Research Council for Complementary Medicine
60 Great Ormond Street
London WC1N 3JF
Tel: 0171 833 8897
Fax: 0171 278 7412

Society for the Promotion of Nutritional Therapy
PO Box 47
Hathfield
East Sussex TN21 8ZX
Tel: 01435 867 007
Fax: 01435 868 033

Society of Homoeopaths
2 Artizan Road
Northampton
Norhamptonshire NN1 4HU
Tel: 01604 21400
Registers non-medically qualified homoeopaths who completed a four year training course followed by one year clinical supervision. Send SAE for list of members.

UK Council for Psychotherapy
Regent's College
Inner Circle
Regent's Park
London NW1 4NS
Tel: 0171 487 7554

Specialist treatment centres

The Ayurvedic Institute
PO Box 23445
Albuquerque
NM 87192-1445
USA
Fax: 505-294-7572

Scott's Natural Health Institute
PO Box 361095
Strongsville
Ohio 44136
Tel: 001 216 238 6930

Yoga for Health Foundation Residential Centre (Courses for CFS(ME))
Ickwell Bury
Northill, nr Biggleswade
Bedfordshire SG218 9EF
Tel: 01767 627271

Supplements and further information

BioCare
Lakeside
180 Lifford Lane
Kings Norton
Birmingham B30 3NT
Tel: 0121 433 3929
Fax: 0121 459 4167
Specialist and quality supplements for CFS(ME) and gut dysbiosis (yeast overgrowth)

The CFIDS Buyers Club
1187 Coast Village Road 1-280
Santa Barbara
CA 93108
Tel: 1-800-366-6056

Clinically Standardized Meditation
PO Box 2280
Bournemouth
Dorset BH9 2ZE
Tel: 01202 518968
Fax: 01202 547444
Tapes and Manuals

International Investigative Dowsing
Alf Riggs
22 Parvills, Parkland Estate
Waltham Abbey
Essex EN9 1QG
Tel: 01992 719735

TriMed
Isis Medical Technology Ltd
The Old Bank Chambers
Town Hall Square
Bexhill on Sea
East Sussex TN40 1QG
Tel: 01424 782626
Fax: 01242 732888

TriMed (Australia)
Jeremy Swallow
SCSI Corporation
Unit 19
No. 9 Hudson Avenue
Castle Hill 2154
NSW
Tel: 0061 2894 6033

TriMed (USA)
Alexander Associates
3700 Lancing Avenue
Colombia
MO 65202
Tel: 001 604 731 7078

Useful further reading

Ali, Dr Majid, *The Canary and Chronic Fatigue*, Life Span Press, US, 1994

Bamforth, Nick, *ME (Chronic Fatigue Syndrome) and the Healer Within*, Souvenir Press, UK, 1993

Berne, Dr Katrina, *Running on Empty*, Bloomsbury, UK, 1992

Borysenko, Joan, *Guilt is the Teacher, Love is the Lesson*, Thorsons, UK, 1995

Brostoff, Dr Jonathan and Gamlin, Linda, *Food Allergy and Intolerance*, Bloomsbury, UK, 1989

Cannon, Geoffrey, *Superbug – Nature's Revenge, Why antibiotics can breed disease*, Virgin, UK, 1995

Carter, Jill and Edwards, Alison, *The Elimination Diet Cookbook*, Element, US & UK, 1997

Carter, Jill and Edwards, Alison, *The Rotation Diet Cookbook*, Element, US & UK, 1997

Chaitow DO MRO, Leon, *Fibromyalgia and Muscle Pain*, Thorsons, UK, 1996

Chaitow, Leon, *Water Therapy*, Thorsons, UK, 1994

Colby, Jane, *ME:The New Plague*, First and Best in Education Ltd, UK, 1996

Collinge MD, William, *Recovering from ME: A Guide to Self-Empowerment*, Souvenir Press, UK, 1993

Couteney, Hazel and Briffa, Dr John, *What's the Alternative*, Boxtree, UK, 1996

Davies, Gwynne, *Overcoming Food Allergies*, Ashgrove Press, UK, 1985

Drake, Jonathan, *Body Know-How: A practical guide to the use of Alexander Technique in everyday life*, Thorsons, UK, 1991

Dries, Jan and Inge, *The New Book of Food Combining*, Element, US & UK, 1998

Gates, Donna, *The Body Ecology Diet*, BED Publications, US, 1995

Jacobs, Gill and Kjaer, Joanna, *Beat Candida Through Diet*,Vermilion, UK, 1997

Jacobs, Gill, *Beat Candida: From Thrush to Chronic Fatigue*, Vermilion, UK, 1996

Kent, Howard, *The Complete Yoga Course*, Headline, UK, 1993

Kermani, Dr Kai, *Autogenic Training*, Souvenir Press, UK, 1990

Lad, Dr Vasant, *Ayurveda: The Science of Self Healing*

Lam Kam Chuen, Master, *The Way of Energy*, Gaia Books Ltd, UK, 1991

LeShan, Lawrence, *How to Meditate*, Crucible/Turnstone Press, US, 1983

Lewith MD, George, Kenyon MD, Julian, and Dowson MD, David, *Allergy and Intolerance*, Green Print, UK, 1992

Macintyre, Dr Anne, *ME: How to Live with it*, Thorsons, UK, 1992

McWhirter, Jane *The Practical Guide to Candida*, All Hallows House Foundation, UK, 1997 (includes a UK directory of complementary practitioners who treat Candida albicans holistically.)

Moss, Jill, *Somebody Help ME*, Sunbow Books, UK, 1995

Shepherd, Charles, *Living with ME*, Cedar, London, 1992

Trattler ND DO, Ross, *Better Health through Natural Healing: How to Get Well without Drugs or Surgery*, Thorsons, UK

Weil, Dr Andrew, *Spontaneous Healing*, Little Brown, US and UK, 1995

Index

BHMA Tapes for Health

*Practical self-help packages designed by
experts to make taking care of yourself easier*

Imagery for Relaxation by Duncan Johnson

Exercises in visualization to help relaxation and influence the functions
of the body and mind. To provide yourself with the opportunity to
learn more about your attitudes and neglected needs. To harness the
forces of the creative mind and change negative attitudes to life.

Getting to Sleep by Ashley Conway

A practical help with insomnia. Promotes relaxation and positive
thinking to put you in touch with your body's 'normal' sleep pattern.

Introduction to Meditation by Dr Sarah Eagger

This tape is a progressive learning programme of meditation exercises.
aching you how to begin using meditation for increasing your peace
mind and well-being.

Coping with Persistent Pain by Dr James Hawkins

Teaches relaxation skills in a greater depth and how to apply those
skills as a coping method during daily activities. To help promote
 one form of involvement into a life of constant pain.

Coping With Stress by Dr David Peters

A programme to teach you how to build the relaxation response into
your life. Understanding stress and dealing with it through relaxation
techniques.

Breathe by Patrick Pietroni

A muscular relaxation technique which explores the connection
between stress and our breathing rhythm. With exercises on how to
control breathing to alleviate symptoms of stress.

Please write to the British Holistic Medical Association at Rowland
Thomas House, Royal Shrewsbury Hospital South, Shrewsbury,
Shropshire, SY3 8XF for full details of tapes and mail-order service.